YOUR JOURNEY
INTO REAL HEALTH

How to Create and Bring Back
the Ultimate Balance Between Mind,
Body and Spiritual Health from Within You

Sanjaya Pandit

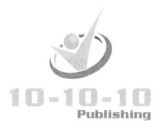

10-10-10
Publishing

Your Journey into Real Health
www.JourneyIntoRealHealth.com
Copyright © 2022 Sanjaya Pandit

Paperback ISBN: 979-8-509458-31-6

Publisher
10-10-10 Publishing
Markham, ON
Canada

Printed in Canada and the United States of America

Contents

To my dad:

*"You died too early in your life and just as I was
getting to know you and all your dreams properly,
so I dedicate this book to you. You had achieved so much
and had so much still to go for. I remember how excited you
were. For me, it remains that I am forever your girl who
had to grow up so fast, and it was the day you left us,
so tragically and suddenly, and which was so painful,
that I realised what life was all about, how precious it is,
and how valuing good health and looking after each
other is the highest purpose, and that everything else
comes from that."*

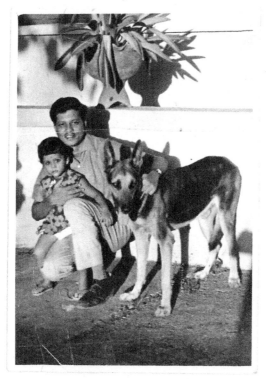

For bonuses go to ...

With thanks and gratitude,

To Mum, for her strength, courage, and resilience she has shown over the years, and the belief she has always had in me. She has been instrumental in supporting both my children and me, and everything we have achieved.

To Dad, for being a remarkable man. Each day, he is missed, but I am reminded of the value of health and being around for my family. He ignored his health to a degree, and put most of his energy into building businesses; probably because he was invincible in his mind. I mean, he was a remarkable sportsman—very fit, agile, and very youthful—and none of us could have ever predicted the ticking bomb that blew up in July 1988, and with it, all his dreams shattered into little pieces. I have never felt as helpless as I did then, when I heard and saw life running away from him, but I understood then that my grief gave me a calling.

To my faith, which for a time was missing; I was angry, and I knew I had to make peace with God for taking away such a remarkable man, father, husband, and friend. I have my faith, and that has always been my ally in life. Every challenge and blessing, whether it be with health, finances, or relationships, my faith has been there all along, and this is why the spiritual part of health is so integral to champion in its various forms. It's not about religion but having the humility to be vulnerable to it.

To my children, Kiran, Ria, Ravi, and Asha, who show me their incredible energy and spirit, and how they live their truth and how they fight for it when someone tries to take it away from them through prejudice, discrimination, and racism, or privilege. They have given me so much meaning, and I learn more from them than anything. I know it has not been easy to have a single mother, and there have been many sacrifices that so many of your friends would otherwise take for granted, so I am very proud of each of you. You are my living legacy.

To the Universe, for giving me a kick every now and again when I forget my mission and cease to look after myself the way I deserve. My drive and intention for good health comes from that, not just for myself but for everyone, no matter who or where you are, or what circumstances you face. We have to help each other.

To all my clients, who have equipped me with so much learning through my work with you, that this book was finally given life. You have allowed me to evolve my coaching and make a difference.

To the Coaching Training Institute and Co-Active Model, for creating a truly divine coaching model that is so intrinsically part of my life. It is simply the best, and it brings out the best in me, and everyone it touches. What a brilliant community of coaches we are.

To my publisher, Raymond Aaron, and his team, who have given me the support to get this book out there.

And finally, to myself, for being a brave and loving woman, parent, daughter, and friend, and for having the strength, resilience, courage, and true knowledge to never give up. I am so very proud of you.

About Sanjaya

Sanjaya is an award-winning lifestyle coach and author. Her experience in the health and wellbeing sector has been extensive, spanning more than a decade of helping people with their health, and to live to their full potential. Her wisdom and transformative ways are unsurpassed, and are facilitated by her deep connection to, and love for, people and nature, involving her wisdom from her own cultural heritage and bringing the dimensions of physical and spiritual being into harmony.

She believes that the agenda of what is good health, has to change. For too long, health has been handled through the wrong focus, making your health someone else's problem. She seeks truth, and requests that for you so that you can empower yourself to work on your health in a wholesome and connected way.

Her wisdom comes from her truth—her dance between illness and wellbeing. She has been through illness a few times, and each time has recovered by using and maintaining the principles in this book. Her drive and reason to help herself comes from the voice that says, "You cannot give what you don't have." That empowers her, even when facing significantly challenging situations for herself and her family.

She never gives up. Her resilience is astonishing once you know her story.

She has a particular authority in the psychological aspects of health, many of which are included in this book. She also has authority in preventing and reversing the global health crisis of today, which is obesity and diabetes, both of which she had to endure in order to learn from it and to connect her truthfully to the discussions and issues of both, for herself as well as other people affected. She, of course, has a scientific background in biochemistry and combined medical sciences.

She is, however, not a lover of too many statistics, and finds quotes far more empowering. She is after a simple thing: to improve your state of being and, therefore, your health from within.

She currently lives in the UK and is working hard to bring all her services online so that she can deliver on her promise, which is to impact the world and request genuine health through her intention and wisdom for the greater good. She intends to continue doing this through her speaking and online platforms, and is currently working on trademarking her new programs that will help you.

Above all, she is a human being, a mother, a daughter, a sister, and a friend, and now a published author.

Foreword

What does health mean to you? Is it just about your physical body, what you look like on the outside, or is it much deeper – a state of being in peace and harmony?

Author Sanjaya Pandit has written *Your Journey into Real Health* to help you connect to your health in a wholesome way, taking elements of your physical and mental health and adding a dimension that is often missed many of the health books you can buy today ... that of emotional and spiritual health.

Sanjaya's wisdom will give you a blueprint to empower yourself by focusing on your health in a genuine way. It gives you the chance to go back to the basics with your health, wherever you are at the present time.

Much of today's healthcare focuses on illness. There are systems that keep you sick, and that has to change if you are going to impact better health for yourself and your children. This book gives you the tools to start those conversations today.

Sanjaya is a credible authority on this topic, because she has suffered illness and restored her own health, without relying on conventional medicine, by intuitively following the principles she shares in this book. She will empower you to take full responsibility for, and ownership of, your health. It is important for you to understand one simple thing: your health is the foundation for everything else you want in your life, including wealth, wonderful relationships, happiness, and liberation.

Raymond Aaron
New York Times Bestselling Author

Health Challenges of Today

Chapter 1
Our Present Day

Matters of Ill Health Today

These days, no one is too far away from hearing news that someone has become ill or has died before their time, through cancer, liver failure, or another lifestyle disease. Equally, we are sharing a life with someone who has a chronic illness. It may be you, and your quality of life is impacted negatively because of it.

The truth is that by just putting our lives on automatic and through warp speed, we don't actually understand the true cost of our own illness or that of our loved ones.

Our growing intelligence, creativity, and innovation has allowed life to be extended beyond belief by advancements in technology and medicine, as well as accessible information that can travel into our homes through the World Wide Web.

There was a time that we could not survive a heart attack, but now, through applying such intelligent advancements, we can keep someone alive for longer, even though the cost to that individual or their loved ones may be greater. It's like half-death and half-life—being kept alive with interventions unnatural to us, and with great compromise. However, I know what I would have given for such measures to keep my father alive for just a little longer. He died at 52 years of age, when I had just graduated. He died of a heart attack.

The term, *chronic illness*, is carried around with us as we go about our functional lives. We give chronic illness the life force and oxygen it needs to thrive, meaning that changes are happening deep inside us that we can't even see; changes that are bringing us eventually to our death, without some having lived a life of their potential at all. In all my years in health and wellbeing, I have not seen and heard from many who have lived life to the fullest. The fact that they have a chronic illness becomes the excuse for everything—a "get out" clause. Instead, we are told to tolerate it, as if that's the only solution. Compromise is better than instant death.

This way of living has stopped many people around the world in their tracks, never realising their full potential; and for those who have eagerly and ignorantly made their material wealth, they have traded it for their health.

There is so much we can now do to stop cancer from spreading, or to even fight a major disease pathway like cardiovascular and diabetes. I partly wish that some of the vast money poured into the research or marketing of drugs goes into rebuilding a better and more lifestyle-based system, rather than one that is heavily reliant on using drugs to treat such diseases. Let's educate and encourage more people in the basics of good health and balanced living. We came into existence with our own natural cures; our body has inherent systems designed to cure and heal us. This may be a simplistic view, but maybe that's what health needs to be again—simple. What do you think?

Today, our natural healing from our bodies is being overstepped and even ignored, for the quick fixes and symptom therapy that today's medicines give us. Imagine being ignored for long enough, not taking up on the gems our bodies have developed since we came into existence. What do you do when you get ignored? It's not nice, and our bodies become disconnected and tired of saying, "I have the answer." Our template for life-optimised, is health-optimised. There has to be more preventative measures put into place.

We like to show our strengths, even though we know at times we cannot be strong. We convince ourselves with coping strategies, and are conditioned into a false perception of strength and pride. I call it the "chin up and let's get going" movement.

I am all for the positive mindset, but if it's tainted with false illusion or even fantasy, it is really not doing a lot good for you or anyone else. As long as we are seen to be doing something, it is good enough.

The irony, however, is that we live longer on managed medications, but as far as we go today, we are sicker as a human race than ever before. What are we all doing to ourselves and to others, when tough statistics show that our children will die before we do! I find that so sad. I am driven to do something about this fact. I want the world to be as disease-free as possible.

We say things like, "We only live once, so why not?" That is what the dialogue is when someone wants one more of anything—beer, cake, sweets, take-out, or that extra slice of pizza to finish off the whole one, eaten by one person alone. Having fun with food and drink is okay, but there are many people who don't take any responsibility for themselves in matters of food intake and health.

From where have we been given permission to drink to the point of incoherence, and to overeat to the point that our bellies are so painfully distended? How is living a lifestyle that breaks all the rules for having a healthy wholesome life, good for us? It is beyond belief. I wonder if we can think instead about taking whole responsibility for our lives, and therefore teaching that to others.

That may just mean that we live a life optimised daily, and go to our death having lived a full life, with the greatest of health. You see, when it's time, it's time. I personally believe that it's written in our fate before we are even given life, and I believe that every human being has a purpose and a reason for their life, something far, far greater than themselves, and our spiritual dimension is to seek it before our time is up. It is like a secret that reveals itself to us as time evolves. I love the unpredictability of death—when it comes, it comes—because it allows me to maximize my life and experience it fully. We don't have old age to look forward to; old age looks forward to us. In saying that, there is much work to do between birth and death. We are on a mission to find ourselves and serve others with our gems. Simply being named by our parents is not our identity, and as much as I like the unpredictability of life, it also energises me to live life with kindness and compassion, and trust and peace.

I want to leave my legacy and walk to the next dimension having known myself fully and having contributed to my world. For that to materialise, I need my health and a wholly synergistic balance between my mind, body, and spirit. I hope this motivates you to look at your life through a different lens, even if you are at the stage where you don't know what you want in life!

So let's be around for many more family birthdays and celebrations by giving ourselves the chance to learn and change what is needed. Stay focused on that by being well, energetic, happy, wholesome, and full of joy and harmony. Let's stop obsessing about how to cheat death, and instead focus on living optimally as a global member of our world community.

When energy is flowing in the wrong trajectory of health, which is the way our health service is sometimes with chronic illness, the measures are not based on lifestyle and root causes of illnesses, but on acute symptomatic relief, and that is not enough anymore. So the way global healthcare is at the moment, it is going to take an additional amount of energy to focus and believe, to bring us back to balance and vitality.

We also know how easy it is to turn a blind eye to all this, never expecting that that person will eventually be challenged to the point that their quality of life is impacted. Furthermore, we react to illness a certain way. If you hear the word *cancer*, people take note. Just look at the masses of charities in support of patients and their carers, and those that are in support of finding cures. And the concern is that with high blood pressure or even diabetes, people don't usually find it that critical; and yet cardiovascular issues remain the number one killer globally!

I would hate for anyone to have cancer, of course; but look at the money thrown into advertising cake sales or fun runs. How much actually goes into finding the cure, when so much of the fundraising monies end up supporting marketing, salaries, and other operational costs for the charity. These are gigantic businesses and, in reality, are hiding behind an ethical and social framework. I would prefer to pay each person directly to better their health, giving them access to green vegetables, education on sugar and its link to obesity and eventually cancer, and information about other food industry misinformation. I have known friends who have spent so much time and energy in supporting cancer charities, only to go home after the fun run and open a bottle of wine and have an unhealthy take away with sugary treats, justifying it with the fact that they did something positive for someone else, or in memory of someone who had lost their life because of cancer. Something is wrong here, don't you think? It's as if people are not connecting the dots; they're waiting for the inevitable before they wake up to preventative ways that can in fact decrease the incidence of death and illness for all of us. No one is immune to cancer.

Many illnesses and what they represent are only the way our media portray the urgency toward possible death, and so it urges action or at least sympathy from people. I say that all illnesses can be dangerous and, in time, will just get worse, because they cannot act in isolation long term. There is always a consequence. It does eventually affect all parts of the body, and that is what we need to realise. If we are only mindful of any minor but repetitive conditions in health, then that is a tell-tale sign to take notice and investigate further. It's called information intelligence from our body, which we no longer comprehend today, but we need to; we overrule the simplicity of body intelligence with a complex and sometimes false mind intelligence.

The deal today is that we put a lot of trust on reactive measures because whilst we have healthcare and pharmacy drugs, then we are okay. I don't think we are. We need to look after each other and hold each other's standards and expectations of self-care, health, and wellbeing higher—much higher than we do today! Why? Because it's our health, and it's a basic foundation upon which everything is built. From experience, health is usually the last thing on people's minds, and the first to be dropped when other urgent matters take hold, which from time to time they do. I know more than anyone how this works. I have spent many years, and what seems like a lifetime, working out how we can have health with everything else.

I mean, it must not be easy to eat well, exercise, and work and play— and yes, there are some who do have the balance—but I am not just referring to health as the amount of exercise and healthy eating that has been so focused on for decades, and to which many aspire, unmatched with reality. The thought of health this way is not enough, but an implementable actionable strategy is the key, but is difficult without a map. I have this map, as I have walked it myself.

There is a way, and the main principles will be covered in this book, with a proven way to get your health set in order to serve you in everything else you desire for your entire, long life. Without it, I am afraid that your foundation on which you build your life is unbalanced and unstable, and things may collapse into a heap around you. It is not to be traded, ever. If you are to live your life in a way that it is meant to be lived—full of joy, laughter, and ease, with an abundance of great things—you need your health with you at all times.

So what is the current state of affairs in our health? It is true that people's perceptions of health for themselves can be different; and by the way, health has different meanings, but for now, assume it is the same basic form. It is also true that very few in the world are at a peak health condition; we tend to think of athletes in that form, but there are others, like elders in our world, whom have lived a very long life, completely disease free, happy, and healthy, so it can be done. Optimal health is when all mechanisms within the body are working together in complete harmony with relative ease. You know and feel it, and your self-awareness about yourself and others goes through the roof; in fact, it's a very enlightening experience living like that.

That does not mean there are no challenges, but it's your reaction to those challenges that contributes to creating and maintaining optimal health. It is possible. It takes motivation.

Sit quietly and think on what health challenges face you or your family members. Are you at your best in health, in your mind and body? And what about your spirit? This book is to cover health at a deeper level, and to start the conversation about health not being a destination or something that can be ticked off, but something that needs attention and work every day; and as time goes by, the relative ease with which you integrate it into your daily life, is stress-free and easy.

Health is the basic foundation for having the truly fulfilling lives that we are given. Let's not waste them. A way to balance health through all three sections of our true selves is the way we need to be living—not leaving health in the hands of physicians, and when we do need to see them, then after not staying compliant with their advice.

I have known people who have been on statins and blood pressure medications, with no improvement in their symptoms; in fact, what the body does is get lazy, and it stops defending itself in the way that it was designed to, which inevitably progresses to higher doses or other ailments of deregulation in the body. We are not meant to be on drugs. The dependency on them means that we are on them a long time before our own bodies eventually give in; and in the meantime, we have lined someone else's pockets.

The majority of today's chronic illnesses can be regulated and decreased, simply by lifestyle measures, and we will only choose that when we decide to take charge of our own health, and stay within the framework where disease cannot get a hold of us, hopefully leaving visits to doctors only for broken bones or acute care. It would be a world without chronic illnesses, surgeries, or the need to write a lifetime of endless, repeated prescriptions.

In reality, I have witnessed and experienced a daily assault on how people, our environment, and our workplaces make it harder for us to be healthy, and make it very easy for us to be sick.

Let's highlight a few examples. One would be our young and the present school or college environment, and how it affects their minds and bodies, and encourages broken spirits. There is a massive increase in children's diseases that would historically have only been seen in an adult, if at all. We now have kids with diabetes, depression, mental illnesses, fatigue, lacking in energy, obesity, and even cancer. As they spend most of their daily lives in school, surely it is important for people around them to be upbeat and positive. What we have is a mix of teachers who either lack the important aspect of having respect for children, or love teaching and recognise their commitment. Teachers in either category are stretched to the point where their health is impacted! How then can they teach and influence kids in a positive manner? No one can give when they are empty themselves. Many in the profession do it as a job, as so many graduates do not get jobs in what they have studied, so they end up in teaching. Their intention may not be aligned with the responsibility and commitment a teacher needs in order to make a difference for every child that is in their class, not just their favourites. Many teachers—and they would never admit it—use language that punishes a child in school, making them feel inadequate and stupid. The problem is that it is difficult to prove, as the system can sometimes close rank.

The school environment for young people is becoming uninspiring, lengthy, and focused on entirely the wrong agenda for their real future. In addition, as if that was not enough, there are some basic needs not being met in a nurturing, unconditional way, like food and feeding times, and exercise and movement.

I work around having regular breaks, with an hour and a half devoted to eating well, drinking water, and getting myself outside for a quick stretch and a walk in the fresh air daily. I do this for myself, yet I feel for my children, who I know are not getting that at their school. Lunches are a mad rush, supervisors don't listen, and pupils get sanctions for going to the toilet and being late back in class because they were last in the lunch queue. Education is all about ill-informed agendas that chase statistics at great cost to children's present and future lives. My kids' school breaks are down from an hour to just under 45 minutes, and they have to queue, get their lunch, eat, go out to get fresh air, and be back on time for class; and if they're late by a few minutes, they are not given a chance to explain—it becomes an automatic detention. Why are some teachers (and every school has them) allowed to do this, when they are meant to be a symbol of good communication? I think, for some, the power gets to their ego; they are stuck in a system, churning out and giving autocratic commands to people who cannot and are not allowed to stand up for themselves. It really infuriates me! I find that the school environment is based on false power, low self-esteem, judgement, and critique. The loving, compassionate, and inspiring environment that once was a pleasure to be around, is dwindling.

Individual productivity has been proven to go up if you stay well hydrated, eat well, and get regular breaks with fresh air. My children regularly come home to complain that they tried drinking water from their bottle but were sent out for disruption. You would think, if that was true, then the teachers may mention it to me, but when it comes to parents' evening or reviews, there is not one single mention of disruptive behaviour. Our educational system is just one area where health and wellbeing are rubbish, because it is a system entirely focused on churning out people ready to work the 9–5 grind.

Despite pressure to get schools to serve healthier lunches, they are still serving tasteless pasta, cakes, and other refined carbohydrate and sugar-laden foods and drinks, and at premium prices. Kids are allowed to drink water at lunch time, where there is a scramble for water jets and an urgent ushering of children away from corridors into the playground. There is no chance to eat properly and no time to get hydrated either. It's a constant conveyor belt. You would be naive to think that the impact on children's wellbeing is a good one. The whole system is against the best of health and wellness for each individual. Teachers spend too much time and energy thinking about how stressful it is, and they don't give their best. I say get over yourselves, and do the best you can, and remember why you went into the profession. If you don't enjoy it, do the kids a favour and leave. Your health will improve, and that will have consequences elsewhere. I have some teacher friends, and listening to their constant whining about the kids at their school, or other teachers, or the new government policies destroying this and that for them, is draining energetically; but they are so attached to their moaning that they can't see a way out or talk about anything else. Are these teachers not taking full responsibility for their time in teaching?

The systematic degradation in our schooling environment results in the detriment of all areas of health within a child's mind, body, and spirit.

Today, school children are either tired, lacking in energy, or they're dizzy with unproductive energy—almost anxious, actually. We have a crisis with mental health, bullying, and self-harm in our younger generation. That's a sign that things are out of balance, and appropriate and progressive change is needed and is instrumental for their future. That means changing the whole system and starting at the basics! It's huge and such a big deal, but the opportunity is fantastic. I for one would like my name on this type of change; it is very much part of my mission.

Luckily, I still have tremendous faith in those teachers all around the world, who do an incredible job for us all. Let's take a minute to appreciate their commitment. They are professionals who have it hard but are ruthless in their commitment to service our young; and if these teachers can make it a happier and more harmonious environment of learning, then there is hope. It is vital that we get this part of their lives right, to serve them their entire lives.

Children will learn more from people and how they are than they will ever learn through a science class or a subject on Hitler. I know many people who "know it all"; they are academically educated but are sometimes amongst the saddest and most vulnerable in our society. In service of balance, there are some exceptional teachers and some exceptional schools, and we need to learn from these environments for other schools. Make each other accountable to improvements; it`s going to take a lot more than raising funds for a new computer.

Another environment that breeds illness is our hospitals, where the sick go to heal. Well, again, having underpaid doctors and staff, with low morale, is hardly a breeding ground for wellness. They cannot and do not have the right infrastructure to protect their health: long hours, red tape, politics, and canteens serving food stuck in the dark ages. There are simply not enough vegan, vegetarian, or good meat choices. You may see a few green apples here and there, but overall, we still need to be supplying canteens with better food. It is, after all, an environment for healing; and hardworking NHS workforces require good food.

I know that such staff always have a choice; they can get themselves organised and pack a lunch that is full of healthy ingredients. And if you yourself are serious about food that you get from a canteen, you would think that the moaning would stop, and you would ensure that you have good food to perform with, but I know that sometimes that is not possible due to such long hours.

There are many organisations that have no real regard for their staff's health and wellbeing; like schools, where they only encourage productivity at a maximum, when the person is consistently only half productive and burnt out. I am amazed at the sacrifices people make in order to look good in front of their bosses; they put themselves in compromising positions repeatedly, with their own sanity and health. Owners and board members do not incentivise and create an environment for healthy workplaces in any remarkable manner. It's all a little too piecemeal, and a tick box, lip service exercise. They may bring an outside consultant who identifies that seating chairs need to change to give better posture; and yes, okay, that's welcome, but what else? What about spaces to have lunch, time to be allowed to walk and stretch, offices that encourage natural lighting, and companies that partner with health organisations to keep their staff well and fit in a dedicated and meaningful way? We are aware of the theory that happy, healthy staff, in any organisation, at all levels, give happy, healthy profits. They become unstoppable in the production capacity, and become a genuine asset. Unhealthy staff are a fault line. Organisations need to take FULL responsibility for their staff in-house, having a dedicated team of professionals on tap to allow for anyone to be seen. In saying that, I am also hearing and seeing that the tide is changing and staff are becoming more receptive to getting help in their workplace on various issues with personal health. However, we still see how working through lunch is encouraged. In-house canteens are no better than hospital canteens.

Another concept that has now become counterproductive is one where workers, who are parents, carers, or those with other responsibilities, are given grace of flexi-working or part time. The problem is that the workload these types of jobs have, is where they still have full time responsibility and tasks, without the pay.

Obligations to the company are in the small print, and so, for many, they cannot be as productive when on a catch-up mission. Anyone in this position leaves the building tired and dehydrated, and not physically ready to start another personal shift of looking after children or a person in their care. For many, they finally stop late in the evening, and finally get some "me" time, usually devoted to overeating and drinking, and watching mundane TV. That is what they do every single day. No wonder they can feel that they are stuck in some sort of time warp.

Actually, this is what many people today feel like resorting to: unhealthier packaged meals and the pleasure of sugary or savoury snacks. That's not food but a mix of artificial chemicals and additives. Many people go back home from work to start another shift looking after their home, children, and husband or wife, and this results in people feeling tired. So what becomes reasonable is to cut corners by buying packaged food, and using quick-fix, stress-relieving strategies, like opening up a bottle of wine. You can hear that loud "ahhhhhhhhh!" when you take the first sip to anaesthetise the exhaustion. Let us instead enjoy wine for the right reasons, because it`s only through an intentional choice that we truly are paying attention to our ways, and enjoying our choices in that given moment.

Health and wellbeing for each one of us can be easily traded for academic ability, savings, and financial and "time" profits. Let's stop this collective habit in ourselves and in other people by showing them how it's done, and instead preserve our life, health, and wellbeing. This way, we each get to live our life to its fullest and its best, and with as many amazing experiences as we can fit in. A life packed full of life is the life I want for you, and the only way is to have full health on your side.

Question for you:
"What impacts your health in an unhelpful way?"

Guiding principle:
"The way of the world today and its teaching
is not giving the best health."

Does Society Let Us Down?

We are fast becoming a race "in denial," and we simply don't challenge each other or encourage each other to be better and to grow in ourselves. Instead, when we don't like something, we complain, moan, and speak behind each other's backs; we steer toward gossip rather than speak our truth. Own up to your dissatisfaction, and instead progress toward reform and recreation; collaborate and give feedback for service of better ways. Just as we are more aware of our oneness in body, mind, and spirit, we are also connected to people all around the world. It does not matter that we have not met or may never meet; we are one species, and at the moment are hell bent on destroying each other rather than helping and building each other up in every way we can—AND WE CAN! I am also talking about the way we go about our daily lives.

Most people skirt around the issues of health and wellbeing, and we need to start on ourselves and our immediate environment and locality. I tested one aspect of this for about a month, and I have to say that on average, for every ten people (strangers and some seen before) I came across, there were eight that felt that it was better for them to moan and live in the past. It is so tiring and hard to be upbeat without acknowledgment; our immediate environment is so low in mood. You can have a brimming smile and, still, they won't smile back. I actually look a little weird, because I smile at everyone, no matter who they are or what their age, and I guess the one person that does smile back, or nod to acknowledge, is enough to override the other eight or so. Maybe this was a little unfair as a statistic—it was a grey, gloomy winter's day here in the UK. Would doing this in summer, with the sun shining, have an impact at driving the smile-o-meter a little higher? Do this experiment yourself, and hopefully everyone you come across will smile back—perhaps you live in a happier place than the city I live in? Let me know your experiences.

Imagine living with anyone who finds it so hard to smile? How long can you last before you join in? We have become too afraid to voice our concerns in fear of not being liked or being rude. If you can save someone's life or give it an amazing quality, I don't think they would mind, as long as they trust and like you. Our relationships need to be grounded in trust and faith, so start conversations with them around how they are feeling and what their dreams are. They may be resistant because their skeptic side rears its ugly head, but persevere, and every time they go back to their default moaning and groaning, give them a hand to see good in all things. In fact, positioning yourself as a lighthearted, energetic, and happy individual is the best thing you can do for others. Those ready to be the same will come and be in your circle.

Most people have buried their dreams so long ago that their present reality is nothing but illusions of the past, which can result in disillusionment on how and why they have not got what they wanted, and how they failed in life. They convince themselves that things came in the way of their true desires. There is always something or someone to blame. These thoughts and beliefs drive their emotions and actions every day; it is like a record playing in the background that we can't hear, but they know how to amplify it when it suits them. That is usually just fear. Seriously, is that what they deserve, and for that matter, do we deserve to be associated with that person? Can we get that firecracker up their backside again so that they can live on the edge rather than in a safe and knowingly uncomfortable place?

Our true selves are becoming dissolved; we mind our business too much, and we are so disconnected with each other that we don't even know what we do every day with our lives. It takes an awful lot of time for trust to be built with each other, and there is so much skepticism with each other's motives. That is not where I want to be; how about you? Forget the people who do not want to know you for real, but concentrate on a small circle of intimate friends and relatives. Start there, and you will attract others to join.

I remember working with a father who was so concerned for his daughter but could not bring himself to say anything to her about her weight, her unhealthy eating, and general mood. She suffered from depression, linked to her weight, every day. She was overweight by 21 stone, and because he loved her so much, he did not want to hurt her anymore; he felt she was hurting anyway. He also wanted to protect her from feeling bad about herself. Of course, as a parent, I know how that feels. He kept quiet, witnessing her deterioration each day, and witnessing her shutting down more and more. He convinced himself that their relationship would become worse than it was if he said anything. He was crippled with the fear of letting her down just by simply encouraging her to become healthier and tackle her issues, even though that was his intuition. Regrettably, he didn't, and this went on for four years. She died, and he knew then, in that moment, that he would never get a chance to change that, ever! On reflection, he told me that the regret was far worse than the fear that he had of hurting her, and he wished he could turn the clock back; that's when he came to see me.

He wished for that time again, so that he could be brave enough to say to her that she needs to get help, and actually for him to reach for help for himself. You see, there is a point where we all become so obsessed with our own worlds that we disconnect from people and let fear get a grip. We all need to protect ourselves from ourselves, and instead have the freedom and conviction to have such courageous conversations. We instead stop listening, stop laughing together, and stop having intimate conversation about life with each other. Feeling lonely and isolated and withdrawn is the worst feeling in the world. It is the true demise of our human spirit. She died of natural causes; she quietly slipped away, and sometimes that's worse than having a reason like a heart attack or cancer. From what Paul told me of her last few years, her body was not coping; but more importantly, her spirit was broken, and there was no will to live and fight. It was too much, and too big to fix.

If we only tackle health with what we eat and how much exercise we have to do, then what would you say to this girl and her father? it is not enough to get fit, or to do with positivity or even mental health; it's about meaning and being in love with yourself, and what you are here to be and do for others. It is a far-reaching spiritual dimension that transcends even religious ideals, and so much of this gets overlooked.

Let's pay attention to each other. Give each other our absolute unbiased attention, listen without the burning need to say words and respond, understand without judgement, and do this regularly every day. You will see the benefits of the relationship in front of you blossoming; and the feeling of togetherness and inclusivity is just awesome. Let's work toward "courageous conversations," rather than superficial, convenient banter.

Practice is where the skill building starts. Many of the principles I share are based on my coaching principles and experience in the health and wellness area for over 15 years; and of course, my own personal life, which is blessed, but it has not been easy. When you use them, you get better at them. Your life will have a bigger and better meaning, and you will witness how quickly it jumps to levels you could only wish for today. It happens, and it's truly transformational.

Let's not let fear dictate our ability to change something for ourselves or for someone else—just have a go!

Don't get attached to the results!

Unfortunately for Paul, he will never know how she felt about his lack of attention; but what I do know is that children expect their parents to be authentic, courageous, and brave, and show them the way in times of need. It is his regret that he could not get out of his own way to help her and save her from herself. Sometimes it's the silent killer—the emotional trauma, the withdrawal from living—that can end it for someone. We have to have the responsibility to make our ONE life be of greatness and meaning, and to use it to help others in every way that we can.

She is at peace, not knowing what impact her absence would have had on Paul, her friends, and other family members.

In his own words, he said, "Perhaps if I had just examined how scared I was for her and her life, and if I had been there to help her in whatever way I could—pay for counselling, help her lose excess weight, or anything—perhaps she would have been able to fight for herself, and she would still be here today."

He knows how precious life is, and so he lives it with vigour and vitality every day, and if he can help someone to lead a healthier life, he now tells them without worrying about what they think of him.

Being judged and misinterpreted is so common in today's society, and we have all created a world where two-way communication is becoming a thing of the past. I love people, and I love communication—talking and laughing face to face with people or over the phone. Our relational platforms are being disrupted through the pressure of "Likes" in social media, but these can muster false relationships, and can never replace the ones in front of you. The concern is for our younger generation, who have grown up with parents who are also on Facebook or Snapchat, and don't know how to hold a conversation face to face or even on the phone. It becomes so difficult to gauge if they are truly grounded.

Our perception is that it's popular to have lots of friends. It's the quantity of people that seems the focus rather than the quality of our relationships. Because of the pressure to be popular, we are actually developing more superficial friendships and attachments than ever before, and the kinds of relationships that are deeper and more meaningful are not so easy to come by. People are more skeptical, untrusting, and guarded than ever before. Good quality relationships need consistency, effort, and authenticity; we cannot truly get that on social media platforms. We can even schedule our posts with a machine, just to keep visible. It is only when there is a deep feeling of safety and trust that someone can be their best and reach their potential in life. It is the function of any good relationship to grow that person and grow with them.

I am not from a generation that grew up with social media. Our mobile devices looked like big hefty bricks, and there was no internet; and yet today, I embrace what that does for us all, and it gives me connections all over the world with interesting people, but I would never replace it with people I know and trust that are with me nearby. For business, it's brilliant, and it has changed many businesses that may have struggled in the conventional way. I am all for learning and new ideas, within reason.

It is not surprising how many live their lives simply "functioning," and the need for us to "escape" from our daily lives seems to be becoming more important and urgent. I think this is a great thing, and it's a start, but doing things in a disjointed way cannot be sustainable. The health and wellbeing space has such a grand mix of conventional and holistic ways, each capturing and nurturing important aspects of our whole selves—mind, body, and spirit. We all have so much access to information for this and that, that actually that in itself is contributing to our illnesses globally. Our pace of life is ever faster than our bodies and minds can withstand. Our brains are overstimulated, and this leads to confusion, fatigue, and brain fog.

We have choices every single day, and it is us that create our world. Doing important work on yourself to get clear as to what you want in your life, is paramount.

There are always choices in everything we experience, from the day we are born to the time we die. Do something better that serves you, and create your way of life.

When we live in a society that does not encourage individual greatness and true potential, it is even more important that you know yours.

Question for you:
"What is your truth,
and is it being compromised in your life?"

Guiding principle:
"Strive to better your whole health first;
then help others for theirs."

What's Expected of Us?

The root of the problems we all face is that we have become unbalanced in our health and are in denial of its true form. It is important to note that there is no perfect balance, and the state of balance or imbalance is individual and unique to you. However, some of you know that something is amiss, and you convince yourself that you will do something about it tomorrow, when you also know that tomorrow may never come, particularly in regard to your health. We have been taught from a young age about career, education, social friendships, money, and so on, but very rarely does the language of true health take priority. It's something we sort of stumble onto when things go wrong, and even then, we take ill health, aches and pains, and general malaise in our stride, justifying hard work or other logical excuses for its presence. How long do we wait until we can't wait anymore?

We are able to do more nowadays due to technology, knowledge, and skills. We pack so much more in as we chase time rather than re-negotiating it. We find it difficult to just be, stop, gather, and acknowledge and grow from this place. Rather, we are expected to be everything to everyone. That's a huge deal for anyone, no matter how confident or strong you are. In time, we are burnt out and too proud to say so, because we have carved our way into unrealistic and unbalanced expectations of ourselves, our functionality, and what we can give to others. We have made an expectation of ourselves to others, and must keep up the performance or charade. Worse still is that we carry out our identity in this way, with the "I am strong enough to cope with anything" type of fantasy.

However, when this type of identity begins to show signs of weakness, you reinforce that belief about yourself, making it stronger and more absolute. In time, it can become cumbersome and unrealistic, but obligations to this fantasy of yourself become a duty. So it overspills into other areas of your life too, taking you away from connecting with your simple human self that is allowed to show some vulnerability. It's like wearing a suit of armour made of steel or iron; slowly but surely, you will start to see and feel its weight on you. That's when resentment can set it, and you can start blaming all situations that demand your strength. You start attracting situations and people where you need to be strong, because this belief is the driver to your thoughts, emotions, and actions, and you unconsciously gather evidence to match it.

What once felt so empowering becomes disempowering, and this resentment of your experiences of late start to play havoc on your physical body and your emotions. It creates a fight between your devil and angel self-talk and behaviour. You do no harm to anyone but yourself; and in time, disease starts to manifest as the disharmony extends to all parts of yourself.

Now you have a problem that becomes urgent, and you need to take note and deal with it. Remember, this book has been written for you to stop this, and instead look at ways to prevent this by being so in tune with your basic and higher needs for health, that it does not pose a disability. Prevention is by far the smarter way of living—living that is connected and authentic.

We need to challenge and stimulate discussions, and design alliances that serve us all, by engaging and really listening to each other. We all have signs of formative disease from time to time, and if ignored, it gets louder and more prominent, just like a child not being paid appropriate attention to. Just then, that child will start to get disruptive as their craving for attention becomes urgent. Our bodies and minds are the same. We need to pay attention and deal with what information is coming our way, or problems will show themselves.

We can take in mixed messages, and also give out mixed messages. It is the role of media and social influence, from family and friends, organisations, food industry-led influences, as well as the health and fitness industry.

Excess information and unqualified trends have one purpose: to get as much revenue as they can. Some people, in health and wellness, have good intentions and have the knowledge to champion change, and are seen having to fight to reclaim people who are lost in misinformation. People are influenced by their thoughts of buying something on their terms, and for that to happen, relation building is paramount. If that does not happen, and all we get is a constant barrage of unnecessary and biased information, we actually switch off. That may be a shame, because I have met many people in this industry of health and self-development, who are really good and have all the right intentions, knowledge, products, and services, but have no interest or expertise in how to market themselves to the masses, or have the funds to do it; but what they do possess are real gems that will transform you. You see, some people are brilliant at marketing and their own PR, but when you get to know them, they have little substance, depth, and breadth of experience and knowledge necessary to help you, although they have a huge following. People are crazy about celebrity status and will do anything to be connected to that whole fantasy, and there becomes a fine line between using that fame to push stuff. They can become self-obsessed and stubborn.

I want to see, instead, an exceptional quality of people having a stage where they can impart their knowledge and authority in the matter of health, and share brilliant content and implementation tools to transform people in their health. Those are who I associate myself with, and who I am looking for to share the stage with. Creating change this way is more meaningful and congruent. Let's all be proactive in our approach to what and who we invite in our circle of influence, including working on the better versions of ourselves. Without visibility and genuine help from like-minded people, it is harder to reach you and do my work. I have to learn these tricks without trading, whilst staying congruent to the reason I want to help. Marketing myself, and putting myself out there, does not come naturally. It's not that I lack confidence or knowledge; in fact, I am incredibly resourceful and strong, but I guess it's my culture and upbringing. We were never taught to bring attention to ourselves or leverage interest in this way, but I also know that some of these ways are the only ways I am going to gain larger visibility and, therefore, be able to influence and change people's health for the better. My intention for a healthier world is pure.

Just as performance-driven targets are encouraged at work, this way of thinking is also spread into our personal and social lives: being the one that is recognised as the best at a party, being the best dressed, having the best car, huge house, and so on. We also fight to be the one that puts on the best wedding or Christmas lights nowadays! This is all to the detriment of what really matters in the end, to each of us, at the end of the day. It's the show, the performance, the facade that people seem to be more interested in, rather than the real deal, and we are all hooked to some degree on consumerism. Look at the beauty industry. People are happy to paste on plastics and chemicals, and when given an alternative that is paraben and phthalate free, natural and ethical, and actually more effective due to scientific innovation, they walk the other way with maximum skepticism. They are the ones that have fallen foul to the million-dollar marketing strategies that the beauty industry uses. Well, if they have money to put into marketing, then they are probably not using great ingredients.

Let's face it, marketing experts can use tricks to sell and glorify hardware nails, when all nails do the same job. The real skill is in the workmanship. No wonder we feel so much more pressure and the feeling that we are not good enough. It's detrimental. It's no longer astonishing to know famous people who seem, in the media, to have it all but suffer great challenges and even commit suicide. It's easier to say that they did that to themselves; but we, as a collective, give it permission because we want perfection. We want people to have it all together at all times. We demand fantasy and media hype, and therefore encourage instability. We are just as much to blame for each other's illnesses as the individual is. There was a time when I was also like this, influenced by peer pressure and how my colleagues were doing compared to me; and I am so glad, through my own personal development journey, insight, reflection, and courageous conversations with coaches, that I was awakened earlier than later.

Our health and wellbeing are simply traded for longer working hours so that we can continue living up to expectations. We all have our version of what good living is, but we need individuals to thrive so that they can make great purposeful contributions to our wider world. We need to be vigilant with our health, and when there are signs that it is deteriorating, we need to choose to quickly evaluate how we can rebalance. It is simply finding a strategy to rebalance what works for you, and do it often, especially when signals show up that suggest imbalances.

We are hardwired into thinking that we need to work hard, earn lots of money, and chase careers to be successful, and not be open to help when we need it, because it shows weakness. As a coach, I am all for living your dream life, but not if it costs you in some other way. No, no, no; there is a way, and I have lived it for many years, completely reversing my diabetes whilst parenting and owning multiple businesses with profits. I believe that you can have health alongside everything else important to you. It does not have to be a compromise, which for many, it is, and has been. I see it in entrepreneurs, solopreneurs, and other skilled and gifted people. They are taught that their business objectives have to be so laser focused that nothing else matters. What's the point of laser focus when other things fall apart in the meantime, and by the time you achieve what you had been running after, you return to the rest of your life, wanting to celebrate, and then find that nothing is the same? You have lost the people that you were so fired up for, your relationships have devalued, and you have lost a little of yourself in the same process, and affected your health in a way that is going to take time and effort to restore; but by now, your empire is going so great that you dare not take your eyes off it, because that too may collapse, and then you would have nothing. You see, now you have compromised choices, and you don't need to get to this point.

Most of this happens because we don't expect it, and we don't listen to the alarms going off when we are so razor focused. It does not penetrate this kind of mindset. So how can this be a best serving principle to be razor focused? That's what entrepreneurs and millionaires will tell you: You have to be razor sharp with focus. Personally, I think this is a male energy, and I find that we can tame it down and still achieve everything we set out to, without compromising our health and relationships. Do men lack that self-nurturing that they so badly need for themselves? I am certainly very mindful that my son grows up knowing his full personal resources and love for himself, without the baggage of gender bias and expectations. Women know about self-love and nurturing—that's their archaic role—whereas men are still conditioned to be looking after their family and getting on with accumulating material wealth, money, and investments. Sickness exists in rich and poor people, and in the middle class. It has no boundaries to age, class, religion, or culture. It just shows up in different ways.

So, it is time for you to think of yourself right now. What's expected of you, by others and by yourself?

What would you like to change, if anything?

How, where, and when is your better and more authentic self present? What do you notice when you are being yourself?

Question for you:
"What do you expect of yourself
when it comes to your health?"

Guiding principle:
"You cannot be everything to everyone
without being that way with yourself;
then and only then, you may decide your priorities."

Limited or Limitless Resource of Time?

I am sure that you have heard excuses like, "I don't have time to eat properly," or "I don't have time to exercise." These are the most common excuses when talking about health goals. There are many more, and as a coach, I can of course empathise with your present reality. It is, however, created by your past thoughts and actions, or inactions. There are many like you, and the frustrating thing is, like them, how can you justify that you don't have time to eat properly? Or that you don't have time to exercise?

Think what else is being justified here! Is it really the lack of time or the lack of respect and self-care for yourself? Eating for biological and nutritional purposes is a basic need, and yet people nowadays seem to be wanting the higher needs without having these basics in a grounded place. You will have heard of Maslow's hierarchy of needs: a system for human needs, a layer at a time. Food and water are as basic as it's going to get, but today we seem to be struggling to put this into a helpful routine.

It's true that we tend to live a full life, where the number of hours just don't seem to be enough to get everything done in a day. It's also true that our lives are packed full of things that mean a lot to us, and time can easily slip away. I do ask myself what I did today that was for pure pleasure and joy, and what was productive, including service in terms of moving my clients further and deeper toward changing their lives. I ask myself how I looked after myself and my family, and how much exercise or movement I had. I also make sure, the best I can, that I meditate and am as mindful as I can be by checking in with my own health daily. I correct minor imbalances that I witness. The one that does get me is my posture at my desk and whilst on my computer. My neck and shoulders can start to hurt a bit, and when I feel that, I stop and reposition myself. I stretch and have a break—whatever I need to do before it becomes a problem.

My self-care is important to me, so I stop for a few minutes. I don't ignore it and wait it out until I can go home and do it then. It is guaranteed that all it takes is 2 minutes of correction at the relevant time, instead of allowing it to go further by typing for another hour or more, making it just get worse.

Now, all of this is in harmony; there is enough confidence and a powerful intunement to get the best of my day, and within a balancing spectrum. It took me years to get to this level of harmony, and people do ask me how I do it. I am not Superwoman; I don't have to be. I don't think anyone has to be a superhero, but people make out that they are so far stretched with things in life that they just make excuses, and earning money will always be more of a priority than health. It has to be the other way around. My programmes are designed with this in mind, and so transitions for you are a step- by-step process, and can be integrated into your new and unique way of living, keeping the good bits and ditching the unhelpful habits.

The point I am making is that we all have time, and it's really about renegotiating it for what we want to get out of our day. Too many people let others borrow their time. It's not theirs—the 9 to 5 working day doesn't belong to them—it belongs to their boss or the company they work for. I hear that time is not as flexible for those people as it is for me, because I work for myself and can choose what I do with my time.

I get the dilemma for those who are stuck in this cycle of working all day, coming home, sleeping, and going back to work—it is a relentless cycle, and very few actually find that they can break away from it. You hear the stories of people who come from London and go to a more rural, natural place that will be better for their family life than the fast-paced business life that London absorbs you into, but you don't have to make such drastic changes to get balance. It's not about all or nothing.

Having worked with people in organisations, who are seeking that magical work/life balance, what I found was that they do not actually take breaks given to them by law; instead, they continue working at their desks. Not only that, but all they have with them is a drawer full of unhealthy goodies. This is deadly serious, as this allows for distractive eating, which can lead to overeating, and these types of foods can give a you a boost in energy but leave you nutritionally compromised and deficient whilst packing in the calories. Anyone can keep going with their work when they have such a boost in false energy, but it is all done mindlessly.

In time, this will contribute to exhaustion, paving the way to a downward spiral to your health. That is just one scenario; another is executives missing out big time on feeding and watering themselves, and taking breaks from the compulsion of back-to-back meetings, without even a breath or time to check if they are okay. Many start their day without a good breakfast and hydration; instead, they keep going on coffee.

We are talking about how you use your time. Funnily enough, the excuses that people make about "no time" takes up more time rather than just doing it, whatever it is. That's the irony. We are procrastinators when it comes to our health, and it has to be urgent for us to give it time. It is a big ask for your body, because it is so patient and is busy trying to bring balance and deal with whatever. Our minds can override any unhealthy signals our bodies give, so our minds can lie to us, but our bodies do not. Listen to your body.

So, you see, there is time, and it is entirely up to you on what you choose to fill it with.

Some people are affected with SAD (seasonal affective disorder), and they find they are more motivated when the sun is shining; so if you are in a place like the UK, then you need to use the right environment and match that with what you set to achieve in that space and time.

There is no one rule here, but it's about creating time and renegotiating the "perception" of the lack of time, filling it with things and people that inspire you and serve you instead, doing together the things you love and which are meaningful. Forget mundane tasks; if they need to be done, choose a 30 -minute window and get them done then, and only then. Most of your day needs to be around your empowerment and putting together progressive building blocks, so that when you do hit the evening lull, there is still more resonating energy in you. I love going to bed tired but fulfilled; my brain has been stimulated correctly, and I go to sleep, full of love for my life, my work, and my loved ones. I get the best sleep, and that's got to be good for my health. I need about 6–8 hours uninterrupted, and then I feel fully restored for another exciting day.

I am saying to you, get out of the automatic pilot mode. We have tons of devices that keep time for us, but real use of time needs to be intuitive. You set your alarm for 6am in the morning, and you find yourself waking refreshed, intuitively, by 5.50am. Look for your individual pattern.

Achieving what you want during the time frame of your day is easy when there are agreed boundaries in place, and the boundaries need to serve you to deliver balance in life. Have a time to eat and cook and prepare wholesome food, and a time out in nature in the sunshine (even though that's a challenge in the UK, since it gets dark at 4pm and is still dark when you awake at 6am). Take time for socially interacting, laughing and having fun, and most importantly, take time for yourself—the wonderful alone time.

There is more and more emphasis on the good feeling that comes from the "Friday" feeling, because for many, it's the end of their work week. In reality, the problem is that you have overspent your hours in work for 5 days, and then have to squeeze everything else in at the weekend. This leads to burnout. I have witnessed exhausted parents and their children, just rolling that way from one week to another. It is not something I would encourage, because that's what your children will follow when they are parents. It's learnt. It's conditioning. To teach them balance, you have to live balance.

Available time belongs to every single one of us, and we can take charge of it.

Let me give you an example of when the perception of the lack of time becomes critically unhelpful. A married business couple regularly said to their children, "Sorry, we don't have time today," which was the normal, consistent response to their children's polite demand for attention and inclusivity. This was for things like wanting to go out to watch a show together, or for something at their school. When the children would get moody about it, and quite rightly show their anger, both parents, who were brilliant at backing each other up, used to explain that the reason they had to work so hard and for such long hours, was because it was important to them, and it allowed them to get the kids all the things they desired, which meant iPads, gadgets, excessive pocket money, and expensive holidays three times a year. It's true that they loved their work, so it was very easy for them to get absorbed into the next big deal to make even more money. They were a really good partnership and business-building team, but they found out the hard way that they were in fact lousy parents. To the outside world, everything was brilliant; they regularly showed off their material wealth, but something sinister and darker was becoming more apparent—their relationship with their children had fallen apart.

You see, children are naturally intuitive and, in my experience, there is no child that would want to ever substitute emotional attachment for any gadget or gizmo. They need to be given the correct and appropriate love and attention. Throwing material gadgets at them is not a sign of love or even kindness—it is a cop out, and a misuse of financial freedom. Children will find any way, even bad ways, to survive and feel important, and without the correct attachment, they may not find their way through life's challenges. They will lack the inner self-regulating resources that are needed to navigate between right and wrong. Well, these children fell into bad ways, but at least with the company they did find, they got to be seen, accepted, and heard, and they felt like they belonged. Drugs, alcohol, and sex were what they became involved in. They were being given lots of money to keep themselves occupied, but their parents had no idea what they were spending their hard-earned money on.

The theory and practice of attachment in its simplistic term is the ability to gain and acknowledge security from a caregiver starting at birth. At this stage it is mostly through a physical dimension through touch and feel, you know the familiar scenario of holding baby and feeding baby with love and admiration when both mum and dad are relaxed and responsive. Then that need to feel and know security continues in a relational setting right to the end of this physical life. From the perspective of the transactional model, it is about the autonomy that says "I am OK and You are OK."

I do elaborate a little more on this if you find yourself curious at all. Please visit www.SanjayaPandit.com and through my next book *Ice Cream or Green Beans*.

Acknowledging and being in tune with your children, no matter what their ages, is paramount, and will cultivate healthy relationships for those involved. Any child, and even adults, love being with others in an easy, authentic, and fun way, and they would swap that for any amount of money coming their way. Their emotional hunger is never satisfied with materials things, and that's the problem. I will go into this again later.

It is so important to have and give recognition, and to have pride and a feeling of belonging in our lives, from the day we are born. These are hallmarks of a long, fulfilled life, and are just as important as nutrition and movement in our overall health. Having been through parenthood myself, married and then single with kids, I know how important these hallmarks are for myself and my children. We are lucky because we have, together, created a very strong bond, and I am confident and reassured that without my presence in the future, they will always be close and understand the importance of these hallmarks with their own families.

There are always choices in every given second of time. We have time, and lots of it, so be in charge of how and what you spend your time doing and being. Don't sell your time to any parasite. Choose what you do wisely, and with some thought. And on the odd occasion, add a surprise and some spontaneity within your time. It will bring you the biggest smile.

Choose time properly, according to what the most important aspects are for you. Fill it with those, and leave some space for opportunities that are aligned with your visions and goals in life, to drop in. This will call forth some balance and happiness, so that you are living your life rather than feeling that you are being pushed and prodded in directions you don't want to go.

Another symptom of ill health is when we can't relax and have appropriate downtime, which is needed in order to balance and restore. What happens is that when we have been constantly overdoing things, our bodies get used to the adrenalin and cortisol spikes that are prominent during that time. This makes way for chronic stress, where our bodies feel like they are in flight or fight mode all the time. We are not designed to be like this, so asking you to sit somewhere to contemplate or just switch off will feel alien. Many people describe noticing this as an unsettled feeling, boredom, or just the fact that they can't relax. But they know that they need to sit and be still, and when they can't, it gets frustrating, and that's when many people make a detour in search of food and drink to get them into a relaxed state—at least if they have their hands and mouths doing something, then that sensory perception is that they are still doing something: eating. Part of the reason for obesity is inappropriate eating. That's when our bodies are not requiring food, but we need to satisfy the cravings for something—it is another type of "hunger." In this case, it's using food to get into a state of relaxation; whereas without it, it's more difficult.

It's bizarre. Nature's natural pathway to balance you, feels at times more stressful without food to accompany it, and if not this, then they fill it with something else to do rather than balance it by being. Relaxing is difficult, and we witness symptoms of anxiety, and feelings of boredom or sadness, or even guilt about the myriad of things we still have to do. If it can wait, it can. Stop and relax.

We take on too much and get burnt out. I mean, look at the different roles we have in our lives. Time cannot be shortened or stretched; it is what it is. So the only way is to choose how we spend it and with whom. This comes down to renegotiating things that give us pleasure, within some realistic boundaries, and getting rid of the things and people that take up too much of our time, for the wrong reasons. Let me give you another example of a self-employed businesswoman who never had time to work on her business. She was constantly being pulled into the operation of her business, so in time, she had no new or potential future customers, as she did not devote any time consistently to grow her business in terms of ongoing strategies. Yes, you may say she was lucky to have had so many customers, but it took all her time to serve them, and it was her "needy" clients that she described as "vampires."

All her energy got sucked into this group of clients, and she spent 80 percent of her time on 20 percent of this client type. Her majority of clients dried up, and they were the ones that she had needed to keep and work with more. This was a wake-up call, because she understood the consequences to her personal and business life. After considerable reflection and considerable anxiety and ill health, she realised her challenges and mistakes. Luckily, she regrouped and renegotiated what she spends time on. She is back in business again, servicing high value clients that take up so little time, leaving her enough time to work on strategies and leadership, and to relax appropriately every day. Her work is now more effective.

If we can transfer such a principle in many other areas of our lives, we will quickly see a shift for the better.

Question for you:
"What does your daily timeline look like?"

Guiding principle:
"Get this: you have time—it's a matter of
changing your perception of it and using it by doing
what is important and truly meaningful for you."

Our Unhealthy Environment

It is not just our time that is cluttered with the "unwanted"; so is our environment. There is too much noise, and too many things, possessions, stuff, and technology. We are overstimulated every day, and that is one reason why people are scurrying off in droves to retreats and places to escape to! Even our home environment is cluttered. Historically, we would return from work, to a more peaceful environment, which was more spiritual and supported a hub of family members, easily and authentically talking to each other at the dinner table. It is a real struggle now for many, to escape to a quiet place at home. Phones are constantly on, and children are scrolling through Instagram and videos, and every now and again, you think there is some peace and quiet, but you get bursts of digital sounds and scrolling feeds. At one time, my son had an iPad, a television DVD, his phone, and social media channels open, as well as doing some work on his laptop, all at ONCE! That was dealt with and discouraged very quickly, and although it is still not as good as it could be, at least he remembers the interruption I gave him before. He now is more mindful, and tries to find moderation with technology.

I have seen children as young as 6, go up to bed with their iPads, and when Mum goes to check that they are asleep as they need to be, they hide the gadgets under the duvet, to trick parents who are incredibly thankful to get some peace in the house before they themselves retire to bed. Constant exposure to technology is detrimental to our health, and most health experts will tell you to switch things off at a reasonable time before bed. In fact, I have one boundary that is agreed with all parties at home: When we eat dinner or are watching a family show, we are not to bring any devices, apart from our hearts and minds and our voices, to the table, so that we can eat mindfully and be together. It gets us reunited, and we love planning and talking about our wishes and dreams and birthdays or particular events that we could go to as a family. This gets us all excited and wishful. It is also good to encourage them to turn their phones off completely, say every Sunday. It is both restorative and balancing.

Lead by example, and show them that their life won't suddenly fall apart because they have not responded to a text on Snapchat!

This practice has had far reaching benefit to my health and quality of sleep. Try it, and see for yourself. It really makes me less grouchy and overtired. It has a magical effect on my hormonal son, who quite likes his mum this way!

Our home environment is so important. It is an area we can greatly influence to be peaceful, restorative, and rebalancing—a place to just be! Now I know and respect that our homes are very personal to us, and how we decorate them is personal. How we use their space is also personal and allows choice.

For many, our homes are open to family and friends, and for entertaining, and that's all great and very important for health, to have a social network. Choose then also to have one room where you can escape to rest that is not always your bedroom. Pick a spot where you can just be your true self.

I know, for most of us, home means so much, and it's heartbreaking to think that it is not the same for everyone. If that is you, find somewhere you can be your true self—a special bench in a wild field, or under a tree, or even in the shed—somewhere that you can make it your own and escape daily, even if just for 5 minutes. Fill it with sounds of water, natural light, and positive imagery.

Look also at your outside environment that you experience on a daily basis. How much green space is there around you? What does your drive into work consist of? What's your office environment like? Your desk? Can you clean it up? I encourage putting a green plant on your desk. How about your office block—is it full of artificial light, with very little fresh air coming in through the day, if any at all?

When was the last time you noticed your local high street? Notice the ways that the landscape of marketing, and enticements to get us to walk into a shop and spend our money, seeks us out. Observe how many food outlets, coffee shops, and discount stores there are. Food is everywhere, and even fuel stops are becoming mini markets, taking pride in further marketing unhealthy lifestyles and food to us, to fill gaps in our hunger. The "convenience" of life and foods is making us ill! We are too exposed to food and drink, whilst all we want to do is get a jumper from a clothes shop. This is what is now called an obesogenic environment, where food is tied in with every experience, without the physical body needing food. Eating out is an emotional experience. The standard of our high streets has dwindled, with very unhealthy food being sold, and with low grade convenience goods that everyone seems to think is a bargain. It is, of course, a choice to shop and give these places your custom. The promise of convenience at low prices, fueled by marketing on such products, will cave even the strongest will and the healthiest person if they are constantly exposed to it. This barrage of advertising and offers plays straight to the childlike part of yourself, and you know what happens to children in a sweetie shop. They want it all.

We are being conditioned to buy so much, and very rarely have the time to renegotiate our environment and what we put in it. Happiness depends on a happy, balanced environment, and a positive and fulfilling environment, inside of us and all around us. Purchase whatever makes you happy, but if it becomes clutter and no longer gives you joy, trash it or give it to charity at best. It's not so much that people buy things; I can't imagine anyone buying something they did not want, unless they are addicted to shopping and find reason to fill space, any space.

It is a known fact that overstimulation from the environment we live in can have a detrimental effect on our moods and behaviours. Depending on where you live, it is also a fact that getting ourselves out in nature every day is a wonderful feeling that gives us a positive, heightened feeling of wellbeing. Test it: Go into a supermarket and see the difference when you walk down aisles of packaged unhealthy foods, compared to when you go down the fruit and vegetable aisles— see if you notice a difference in yourself. It's the same as when you are tied to a desk, and then walk out into the sunshine, with nature, the trees, the birds, and nature's beauty.

A cluttered environment can become toxic to us over time, and we have started to suffer from this in physical forms ranging from sleep disorders, headaches, tiredness, lethargy, and lack of energy, to name a few.

Let me pay attention here to our food environment again; there is more and more of a call to spend money on quick fixes. Food and drink are accessible in all ways. For example, "Greggs," here in the UK, is a high street bakery that has just opened up some drive-thrus. So why would you want to stop walking to a typical high street store, and instead drive to get your sandwich and cakes? It was a gap in the market; drive-thrus only belonged to McDonald's and KFC, and with so many people not working in town, many wanted something different—and yes, it filled the gap, and that was clever! But Greggs is not all that healthy either, with most of their products being flour-based savouries or sweets. This leads to the problem that we have for an obesity epidemic. Convenience gives the same problems we have currently in health. We discourage movement and meal planning.

Today, despite all our developments, we have little choice for good food. We pay a premium price for good food and essentials. There is too much processing in the food industry; even fresh produce is wrapped in plastic, and our future generations do not have good enough skills to navigate themselves with better choices for food. Cooking skills have been on the decline because it is not properly taught in schools or at home anymore. Parents are working all hours of the day and night to make ends meet, mixed with all their other duties with children. Cooking from scratch is a dying art in schools, which once was pivotal to balancing the curriculum. I was taught at school as well as at home. Today, cooking classes in schools give out a recipe sheet a day before, and ask children to bring ready-made ingredients shopped for at supermarkets, with a few fresh ingredients like herbs or vegetables, but if they are learning to make a pie, then surely they also need to understand about pastry and how to make it from scratch with different options that spans individual choice. Instead, I am afraid it is about funding and becomes a tick box exercise. We have to bring back staff dedicated to really teaching cooking! The emphasis is on academic skills rather than skills that will give people health, vitality, and longevity. However, all is not lost, and taking full responsibility on what we are willing to learn means we stop moaning and find ways to teach these important aspects for ourselves. It's not about being the best cook or even about a career path to follow; it is about understanding the benefit to you. All is not lost because there is time, and this is a great time to get some aspects back into play. There is a force waking up to the needs, being developed and created through sharing people's stories, health experiences, and functional medicine, where we collectively seek to rebalance and put right what is lost for us today. The future looks much more balanced and positive if we are able to engage people in better ways of being.

What we do today will determine the future of our health.

The rise in energy drink consumption is staggering, as is the decline in mental health. People all over the world are tired and lacking in energy, and live with deep tiredness that one night of good sleep will never cure. Life expectancy for future generations is on the decline; in fact, it is predicted that our young will die earlier than we do. How alarming and sad is that? Each of us is responsible for that. Change can only start with you.

You only have to read about mental health and how it is such a big problem. These problems can be solved and will easily disappear when we take a moment or two, daily, to balance, become more aware of ourselves and our desires, speak the truth, speak for ourselves, and take care of each other as fellow human beings together.

Animals do this in the wild, so why not us? Let's get back to basics with health, feel supported and included, and know our true strengths and areas for growth. Let's connect to a bigger and more diverse community, helping each other with kindness and dignity. A deep sense of belonging in each of us would solve most global social crisis. We have to start somewhere and be accountable for our own world first, before the impact is felt elsewhere. It is when we are not grounded and at ease with ourselves that we start the blame.

To do this, create an environment that nourishes you. Do whatever you have to with your environment that gives you some peace and space to be creative and think better. It means decluttering, and doing it every now and again all around you—in your bedroom, your wardrobe, your office space, your fridge, your car—and even changing your way of shopping from time to time, to make room for better food and drink, and to strive to look at your health and wellbeing needs every day.

I have created a space in my house that is only for me. It is my own space to write, think, dance, or create. It is an inspiring, bright, open space, with a full view of nature's sights, smells, and sounds, which gives me true, simple pleasures. The challenge was to "let go" of some furniture that I was attached to but which was clearly adding to the cluttered feeling. I took a deep breath in and out, and then let it go. I took it to the tip, tipped it over into the big container, and suddenly felt lighter and freer, and there were no negative emotions attached to these pieces—they were just clutter. The sound of it freefalling was so bizarre, but when it hit the bottom with a thud, it was liberating to let go.

Now with the space being decluttered, I can recharge in this space every day, and write and think, and sometimes empty my mind and focus on just "being" there in the moment.

My bedroom was also something I decluttered at the same time, and I have made sure it has no technology and is slightly cooler than the rest of the house, especially an hour before sleeping. It is a peaceful, neutral-coloured space that contributes to my restful sleep every night, so that I am energised for an early start and can make the most of my working day. It's a place where I meditate and acknowledge everything I am grateful for, and I do this once in the morning and once at night. It has given me an immense feeling of happiness, and my clarity of thought has dramatically improved. It has continued to have a massive impact on my work, and together the results are so powerful that even challenges are no longer challenges; I just handle them better.

Question for you:
"What about your environment brings you
true joy and happiness, with that feeling
that you have good health?"

Guiding principle:
"Create the environment around you to be loving, simple,
nurturing, and healthy, and then do what
you need to in order to sustain it."

The Impact of Stressors

Today's worst state of being is "stress," and this state can transform your good physical body into a diseased body, because of the changes it makes to regulatory and otherwise balanced mechanisms in your body and mind. It also affects your mood and spirit, and instead of feeling light, you can feel heavy and burdened. What if we put stress in a bottle and looked at it from outside? What would we see? What does stress smell like or taste like? When we open the lid, would it be a solid mass, or an escaping gas or a liquid? What's the colour we see? These are not trick questions. The point is that stress does not take any physical form unless you allow it to do so in your body, and that is where it can have power to make physical changes to your health if you allow it.

People feel stress in so many different forms and in different places in their bodies. It is created through different experiences, and the way we each deal with it is also very different because it tests our resolve and strength, and how we can think our way through it so that it doesn't get a hold on us. We all have a different threshold for stress, so we have to have varying measures to combat it before it starts to make the changes within our chemistry. I would say that generally, with the way we live today, our thresholds for stress are much lower because our bodies are already out of balance. Thoughts such as, "Oh no, I am going to be so late today, and the boss is going to be so angry," or "I hate the way I look," are some statements that can create stress, because we make unrealistic assumptions and judgements of others and ourselves. We have become clairvoyants, predicting and assuming outcomes to such statements. This is what causes us stress. It is a reaction or an unrealistic view, which makes us think more of the same, getting caught up in a negative loop, with consequences to our health.

Over time, our bodies become alert and sensitised, and the slightest thing can trigger a bigger stress response. I have seen people drop and break a glass at home, and react in a way that was ridiculous and over dramatic. Our reactionary response, therefore, is on auto pilot, without giving us the time to think things through, without just reacting. We also associate a certain emotion to this way of being or thinking, so it does not matter whether a situation triggers off a thought, because it can also trigger emotions.

The hope for people who find themselves in this position every now and again, and for those who are under chronic stress, is that they can make a few small changes to the way they think about situations and worry, thus changing their emotional charge response, and therefore protecting their bodies from negative impacts. Once we know and can do it, we can teach our little ones to do the same, and reach further out to our circles. Stress, these days, is so powerful that we can literally pass this on to each other. Have you ever been in the company of someone who is stressed when you met them, and you were happy and light, but soon after, you also felt that stressed energy transfer, and you started feeling your neck and shoulders tightening up? Well, it got passed on to you!

This is because no one likes anyone going through anything that is stressful for them. We like to help, so we suggest things and calm things down; unfortunately, until they are ready to listen, you will be talking to a brick wall—an over-sensitised state is actually a state of no feeling, as I like to call it. They are not present, aware, or mindful of anything. You have to let them ride the adrenalin wave, and when it dumps them back on land, then there is a chance to talk some sense to them. It would be futile otherwise.

We can be in control of stress and any situation that causes stress to us, by thinking better. Avoidance of dealing with it is counter-productive, as it may give you peace for a few minutes but will haunt you for longer, as it remains unresolved; so fearlessly deal with things head on, and think of these situations in a way that is good. Imagine yourself dealing with it in a way that does not compromise anyone— a win-win at best.

Remember that we are designed for short bursts of stress, so sometimes it can be the very thing that keeps us alive and at optimum performance; whereas so many of us live in our all too familiar comfort zones, not encouraging new things or speaking to people who challenge you. We may not like it, but like I said earlier with the statement, "Get out of your own way," our brains and corresponding physiology welcomes it for our own growth. Our natural mechanism of flight or flight is a stress response. We have it covered; it is only when this gets played out too much that we will start to suffer. We are not designed to be fighting against a sabre tooth tiger every day for 7.5 hours!

What's your current prolonged sabre tooth tiger experiences in life? What's the real impact of it on your current health?

Question for you:
"What are your stressors in your life?"

Guiding principle:
"Stress—do not fear it, just accept it;
let it lose its power over you,
and then change your perspective on it,
remembering that some stress is good for you."

Chapter principle:

"There is a lot going on outside of you to pull and push your health in different directions. To attain health in a balanced way and to sustain it, if you let these external factors influence you, you will find it very difficult. You know how easy it is to blame the environment, lack of time, too many life roles you play, and stress; that is the reality of the present day. I get it; it's not easy, but it's worth it!"

Chapter 2
Misleading Information

Can We Really Trust
Our Government with Our Health?

I believe that having health in its entirety in anyone else's hands is tricky for both parties. In the case of the government, for example, because of size and changing methods and structure, it makes it less possible for transparency and real time knowledge, making new and much needed implementation and accessible informed knowledge hard to come by and untimely. There are many things that are going on behind the scenes that people do not know about, and most of them are not in the best interests of the public that they are serving. Many of the influential giants, in food, agriculture, medical and pharmaceutical, finance, business and media, are in collaboration and have reasons to help each other. They hold reigns in place for policies that see their interests protected. This is to the detriment of the rest of us, and sometimes even of the mass of medical and healthcare doctors that simply cannot care for us in the way they want to.

Look at the misguided advice given to all of us about the issue of fats in our diet, and instead eating a low-fat diet, which has been taken up by so many; you cannot go to the supermarket or any weight loss centre that does not regurgitate the same dribble, and yet obesity is on the increase, in adults as well as our children. It is so frustrating that obesity is still not focused on in a way that surpasses diet and exercise models, when we know that it is more complex than that. Nutrition courses and dieticians have the same outdated knowledge as the governance of these courses that rely and have to be in line with government policies. I have not met a single nutritionist and NHS dietician that uses knowledge that is updated or even slightly controversial, not for the sake of their publicity but for the sake of the nation. I am stating this from my experience and the lengthy talks and discussions I have had here in the UK with many clients and patients of these same people. It simply is not enough and does not work.

Now, I know that most healthcare providers want to do the right thing by us, but patients of today have changed, and so have the challenges they bring to nurses and doctors who are either ill-informed or don't have an interest in a more holistic approach to their patients' health. In the last few years, this has improved, with more doctors in primary care really embracing the new path going forward; I encourage you to have a discussion on this basis with your primary doctor. Private healthcare is better to embrace this than healthcare like the NHS. Again, in the UK, it's our NHS doctors who also run private clinics, so there cannot be any new knowledge. These doctors are too busy to learn a new set of skills. Lifestyle medicine, for doctors that are part of any system of healthcare governed centrally, is a new language. I want patients to have a choice in how to look after their health. We still all live with the belief that doctors know best, but they don't, and I don't think that is what they think about themselves either—well, at least if they are not arrogant or have too big of an ego. We get this type of person in any profession. That unconditional trust we have, and more in some cultures, has us conditioned into believing this, and can lead to untruths and a breeding ground for abuse because doctors themselves are stuck between a rock and a hard place.

I applaud doctors and health care workers who put their heads above the line in order of truth.

The question is, how long are you prepared to tolerate this? Public health has a responsibility to inform us, but who says it has to be the truth? Wealth in healthcare has been modelled and created the wrong way, and now we have problems.

There is a way that wellness can be celebrated and encouraged, and wealth redistributed. Instead, the system chugs along, and we are all caught up in it.

Look at the outdated Eatwell Plate here in the UK. Such information includes carbohydrate overload—type 2 diabetics are told to eat carbohydrates to the point that they are frightened if they don't, in case of a diabetic hypo. In their minds, they are frightened to go to sleep at night in case they have one during their sleep. They are literally scared of passing out or even dying. This is the firsthand advice experienced by myself and many in my close family, with diabetes. Thank goodness, I knew better and followed my own guidance from within. The objective is to keep sugar levels steady; but in practice, the Eatwell Plate gives peaks and troughs. Anyway, this also poses another problem: advice and guidance given to diabetics by non-diabetics; and advice on obesity, given by people never having had a weight problem. Yes, the theory may be correct and given with good intentions, but until you live with it and recover from it, you don't really know! This is a dimension of knowledge that has been completely ignored. How is that right? Experience in anything is key, and sharing that is also helpful to others who can relate.

Most people understand carbohydrates as rice and flour-based food, like bread and pasta, which all give a large enough glycaemic load and is poor advice for diabetics; and actually, it is for most of us. Fair enough, athletes can have it because of their energy expenditure and lean muscle mass. But for the rest of us, it is irresponsible. Dare I say it that perhaps they want us sick so that they can control our health? There is very little nutrition in these foods, and usually any food fortified with extra vitamins and minerals means there is not a lot in them. These foods are not supplements; these are regular things we all pick up during our weekly shop. Does that not sound a little misguided to you? Who would you think is behind this advice? When did carbohydrates become essential in our nutrition plan anyway? Fats are essential; in fact, if you don't have essential fats, there is an impact on the absorption and functionality of the fat-soluble vitamins, A, D, E, and K.

Fats in our foods, for so many years, have been part of the bad food group that caused heart disease and obesity, when in fact it was always the processed foods, labelled by the food industry as "low fat." Processed foods have artificial rubbish that manufacturers put in for taste as fillers, including sugars of every variety and form possible. These are cheap ingredients and addictive ingredients that get us hooked to buy more and more, nicely lining the very pockets of the players in the food industry, who are always looking for cheaper ingredients and easier manufacturing capability for maximum profits. Just walk into any supermarket today and have a look for yourself. Look at the ingredient lists. Supermarkets no longer look and smell like places where we can get real food. It is, however, a delight for the nutritionally uneducated people and convenience shoppers. Real food smells fresh and is vibrant in natural colour, but our fresh fruit and vegetables smell of the plastic they are wrapped in. Our meat smells of the packaging. These foods are far removed from their original source, and are picked way too early for any actual nourishment. Our land and water are heavily polluted. Fish are contaminated with mercury. The soil our crops are grown in, is depleted.

It is a stressful experience shopping, having to navigate and find what you want without overspending and getting sucked into all the crap. That's why I try my best to source locally grown produce, and when I do have to go in, I stay at the periphery of the shops: fruit, vegetables, meat, eggs, dairy, and toiletries. The other stuff does not need to be there, but that's where all the profits are, and actually is 80% of the overall stock. These are huge buildings taking up a lot of land. Fresh produce is expensive, but packaged food is cheap, or has most of the deals in order to make us keep buying it. Our bodies do not get nutrition from these foods, and so for those of us who know better about real nutrition that is lacking in today's foods, we look for supplements to get us the complete nutrition we are after—largely the micro-nutrients depleted in our soils—and I may add, the supplement industry is also a little tricky to navigate through. The supplement market is flooded with low, cheap ingredients that actually deliver very little of the nutritional supplement that you want. So be very careful; you may be wasting your money but, the publicity from this is not all that fair to those companies that are absolutely brilliant at making supplements to enhance your health. Take a look at those companies that are making fantastic quality and life-enhancing supplements, and who have credible scientific and evidence-based proof. There are only one or two companies worth considering, and because of the quality, you pay a reasonable price, but the benefit is exponential.

You see, I have observed people in supermarkets, and whilst they don't know it, they are actually buying through stress, from the huge choices and different messages bashing their brains in what to choose. They have to manage their conflicting devil and angel voices—their self-talk, aka chatterbox! And the biggest management issue is their inner child within them; that part of them that is mesmerised by the deals, and all the reductions and discounts, and the nature of the promises on the packages of today's foods—the unhealthy, shiny, packaged stuff that promises all sorts of good things and is marketed to you—such as ice cream, puddings, and pizza deals. And as you age, that inner child still wants some exposure, so it's the alcohol that becomes the next "grown up" thing to do, and the convenience foods. The enticement is the same—those clever marketeers! And if you have a strong and stubborn inner child, it's chaos, and you will buy into the fantasy of all the foods being offered.

Our inner child has been brainwashed by influence and advertising; so it only sees the fantasy of it, and not the actual consequences—it is very clever marketing.

I touched earlier on fats that publicly have a bad reputation, and that are bad for us and cause cardiac problems because of cholesterol issues. This started the partnership between government, public health, the food industry, and the pharmaceutical drug companies. Our foods became saturated with sugar instead, and it remains the biggest untruth that fuels the disease, the obesity, and the mental illness that we now have. Our foods are packed with crap because what would have been better and more essential in fats was substituted with sugar and then tested in taste forums to be palatable and addictive. Stop buying low-fat, processed stuff. If you want low-fat, then eat whole vegetables and fruit; and as fats are essential, choose nuts, seeds, avocados, meat, and oils like coconut and olive oil. Stop buying anything that has processed sugar. If you want sugar, eat whole fruits—not lots of smoothies or juices and dried fruit—like dates or figs, in moderation.

The consequences of the type of food that is available and affordable, are what we are seeing in our declining health and increase in lifestyle-based chronic illnesses. Disease is more prevalent in our populations globally, and is no longer centred on age or getting older. Too many people are on and off diets, and counting calories rather than looking at eating well and being well. Some, having dieted for their entire adult lives, are now having a dysfunctional relationship with themselves and with food, with deteriorating mental health. I will write more about this later.

You know there are populations around the world that live to an incredible age, without disease in areas of mind, body, and spirit, with all three working in harmony. In other parts of the world, like the USA and UK, our adult population, and even children, are sicker than ever before. I shake my head at the statistics of childhood obesity and all the related problems. Why are we even at this stage? We are so far removed from real food, the type that our ancestors and grandparents ate. Instead, we have come to think of packaged and processed convenience foods as the thing that gives us a bit better quality of time. Maybe it does for a short while, and that's why convenience eating and foods have so much exposure. The convenience revolution makes us lazy. It is arguably easier to stuff pre- packaged food into the oven whilst you pour a glass of wine or get about doing some much needed chores around the house, but it's about the reliance that builds to it then. Can you see that?

This unreal food has set about an even bigger problem with our bodies; it affects our balance of gut flora, which have an exemplary job for our healthy long lives. It is by far the single most and complex network of signals and connections to your overall health. If you think about it, our human design is to take in food, and if it is toxic, our bodies deal with it, ending up attacking us instead. We have lost the diversity of our gut flora, which is essential for us to survive in a fast-changing world. Processed foods strip most of the goodness that would be an integral part of real food at its source. That's one of the reasons that manufacturers have to fortify food with added fibre and vitamins and minerals; processing is the part of the manufacturing process that strips it away. Manufacturing processes are also aligned to be for the best interests of profits, so many do not have good manufacturing practices that have our core health in mind. Our gut microbiome needs fibre from our foods; but on average, we only eat about 10–15g a day, if that, which is very low.

The juicing trend is great for people who don't eat fruit or vegetables, but with juicing comes two main problems: Firstly, we have too much fruit in the one helping of juice. You would not ever think of it as having too much fruit when it is meant to be so good for you, but too much of it is not helpful. If you think about it, if we were to have whole fruit instead, we would stop at one or two at best. It is rare that you would eat two apples in one sitting, or two bananas. The juicing, for some people, allows their sugar to spike, and therefore increases insulin secretion to deal with the sugar in your blood, which has to be finely controlled. As it does this, you can feel hungry and crave sugar again. Notice, when you eat a high-sugar and carbohydrate breakfast at 8am in the morning, how hungry you feel by 10am, and you are ready for something like a chocolate or bacon bread roll. This can also lead to problems with weight management, and may put you into a pre-diabetes state if sustained for long, and your body will be sensitised to insulin secretions. Insulin cannot do its work and act in the way it is designed, increasing your risk of full-blown diabetes, inflammation, and other risks. The second is that most of the fibre that is in whole fruit is thrown away by the juicing, and that's what our good, friendly, diverse gut bacteria love to have. Good gut health is key to so many important physiological pathways for our survival and health, including immunity, brain health, and longevity, and has an impact on many of our systems, including brain health, hormonal regulations, and digestive health, which needs to be at peak performance in order to convey the functionality of our food into energy for our cells, and which keeps us alive daily.

The government and public health do, however, have a responsibility to be seen as doing right by us, so we do see many incentives like parks and green spaces, and even the encouragement for swimming, for the family, which is offered for "free," alongside various other physical activities. This is all welcome and creates good public relations as they try to bridge the gap of what's accessible to our poorer communities, as there are many health inequalities. These communities have gaps in their knowledge and education, and therefore are less likely to challenge information. Some can be on supplemental benefit income, and therefore do struggle to make ends meet, let alone pick up good healthy food, as this still costs far more than packaged and tinned food, if we can call that food!

The "free" bit has limited mileage because it misses an integral part of our human change process, and that's motivation. So these incentives fall on deaf ears. The problem we have in the UK is that our NHS is free to access and is actually abused by many. It is becoming paramount in devaluing health, and is making the way we look at health as reactive rather than proactive. Each and every one of us can make our choices aligned with our present and future best self, built around best health. But we chug along and are so concentrated on so many other aspects of life, like careers and education, and money and mortgages for our homes, etc., that we ignore the needs of our own health. The frustrating attitude I come across every day is the view that someone else can sort your health, and that the responsibility for your health lies with someone else. This is ridiculous.

Our own health is our responsibility, and when we have good health and wellbeing, then we share it and champion others to work at it. It has to start with you.

We have become people who like quick fixes without much effort: the instant gratification concept, where if something needs fixing, it has to be done like yesterday. The system encourages doctors to be highly paid pharmacists, and we need to get back toward more functional medicine practice, where doctors take the time to understand the complex issues for their patients, and talk about lifestyle, nutritional, and mindset medicine. They need to partner transparently with holistic practitioners and health coaches, who for years have been doing this exact thing to a group of people that don't believe in pill popping, and are desperate to understand the root of their ill health. They don't want—and nor do I—to "stick a plaster on" therapy.

I have a high regard for our doctors, nurses, and NHS staff, as well as equal respect for my colleagues in functional holistic practice, but no one knows it all, and because each one of us humans is unique and individual, that general advice is not good enough. Writing a prescription is usually targeted at general symptoms, without the true and informed knowledge of the cause or disease process. It is very hit and miss. Collaboration and transparency with patients is key, and sharing knowledge for the better good of everyone is important.

However, I am glad that today we are getting doctors to admit that they don't have all the answers, and to understand that they need to be battling against over prescribing, and instead need to go back to talking more about lifestyle with their patients, and really understanding the underlying causes of disease and symptoms in all their deserving patients. But they also need to partner with independent practitioners, in local areas, that can really help with this.

I have a great relationship with my doctor now, but it wasn't always like that. I, too, used to take this pill and that pill, and it never did anything apart from mask the symptoms. It was only when I looked at what was causing these random and independent bouts of ill health that I started joining the dots and got an understanding of myself, how I work, and what I need. Actually, in truth, I am really grateful that the consultant diabetologist that I once had, said that I would be diabetic for all my life, and that he wanted to increase my prescription in numbers and dosage, keeping me on medications for as long as I live. I was 37 years of age. Was that right or wrong for me? Not once during my consultation did he ask how I was coping, as he knew I had recently had twins, or tell me what I could do that would help my sugars stay lower and more normal despite the fact that I was on meds prescribed by him already. But he did want to prescribe and change my medications to the ones that the pharma rep had just talked to him about, as I had noticed her leaving, and her card and information was on the same medication.

What he did not know was that I had spent many years in the pharmaceutical industry, and I knew how that aspect worked; and of course, in those days, almost 30 years ago now, it had a rather unruly regard of APBI rules. So I challenged him and stated my will and desire to beat diabetes somehow without medications. I did it in 6 months and returned my sugars to a very good normal. That is where I remained for over 17 years—diabetic free and without a single medication. With knowledge and experience, and my coaching, I run clinics to help people prevent, manage, and beat diabetes.

To keep it that way, I have to be proactive rather than reactive, always keeping on top of my health and what information my health and blood results can bring about. People deny themselves that knowledge, which for some can be a risky strategy. Underlying disease does not always show up, but if it is deteriorating, it will show up—that is guaranteed. The question is, will it be too late? This way of responsibility and accountability is what needs to be applauded, not the regular visitors of primary GP surgeries, who just want to moan about this and that, and are usually just full of coughs and colds that cannot be treated anyway and are wasting their time, NHS staff time, and other valuable resources—they are victims of their own plight. I'm not sure why I pay taxes for that attitude (had to be said)!

Our NHS in the UK is at a breaking point, so let's use it to get treatment for acute illnesses, and when it is urgent to see a doctor. Let's try to prevent being ill or developing anything chronic, and take full responsibility for ourselves by living as near a balanced life as is possible, and with health and prevention of disease in its highest regard. Why do we tolerate anything that drains our health service and doesn't do anything to help it?

I can't imagine anyone tolerating this in a private practice. We will only raise our NHS standards if our own standards are raised first. There is no point in just complaining under your breath—your voice matters and needs to be heard.

We all deserve the best experience in correcting our health and staying well.

Sickness and disease no longer just belong to the poor. The rich and middle classes have jumped in too. Whatever, it is about becoming self-motivated and knowledgeable, and taking responsibility individually and collectively.

It is in our own hands to rebalance, restore, and hold each other accountable. It is frustrating that there are people who take their health so much for granted—they drink, smoke, and lead a lifestyle that is so ridiculously unhealthy—all for enjoyment by the way, and it's this population that abuses the generosity of the NHS. Then there are people like me who work hard at keeping healthy, and that are paying for this said population because it is often them who uses up accident and emergency, and uses up resources of the police force through accidental damage whilst intoxicated. Meanwhile, there's a little old lady that has been burgled, and there are no police officers to investigate this in time. We are not here to abuse resources but to ease the burden so that everyone can tap into it when needed, rightfully.

The health care systems around the world are different, and the motivators to keep well are when you know it's expensive to get sick. We will see many people lose their lives first before we are forced to wake up. I am trying to wake you up before it is too late!

If you are only going to look at your health because something goes wrong, and then fix it and then go back to your way of living, guess what! It will come back stronger—much stronger—and there is no system in the world that will fix it, because once you are caught in the net, you will be caught for life. Maybe it will be a life of prescription drugs! What was a little problem becomes bigger and more evident.

So let's take what is offered here and also through our public health, that being in nature is free and is the most restorative. Here in the UK, we can moan about the weather. I prefer a more consistent climate, but I also feel blessed that we have so much beauty and green spaces in the UK. We make use of parks and tennis courts in the summer, and also can have a healthy picnic and just be outdoors taking in the sights and sounds of nature. It always nourishes us wholly.

Choose one thing you can easily do together that will serve your health. This exercise is not about the subject of what you do, but more about doing something and understanding the power of taking responsibility for yourself and for each other, and then moving further by holding each other accountable and doing it consistently if it works and nourishes you.

I have experienced so many people that I could never truly ever count on, and some were members of my close family. If this is the same for you, it needs to change, or you need to get in with a new set of people that you can count on every time, and they on you! First, make as many options as possible, and then take a vote to see what wins for the majority, and set a timeline to engage with this activity for say six months, and make everyone in the group accountable. Let no one down in the group; encourage that this is something we need to be doing consistently to get the results you are seeking. Remember that initially you may all find it exciting, but as time goes on, people start to talk themselves out of it. By each of us in the group taking ownership for ourselves and others, it makes it a very powerful motivator to keep going; so whatever you choose, choose it wisely, and not on a whim. Have fun with it, and reward yourselves in healthy, appropriate ways each week that you all do it.

Question for you:
"What do you see about your health
that is someone else's responsibility? Be truthful!"

Guiding principle:
"Only you can help yourself; you may not have all the answers,
but they will come in time. Help yourself in your health—it's time."

Is the Information You Get Factual or a Myth?

Having spent so much of my life so far in health and wellbeing, I have come to realise the common excuses stopping people from getting to where they want in their health. This is fueled by marketing, misleading information, general confusion, and the increasingly larger dieting industry messages. We want people and programmes to fix things and solve things for us that are hard for us to solve ourselves, so we are continuously on the lookout for this type of help—quick fixes and effortless transformation, where the work done by someone else and something else is always more attractive.

This gives birth to many of today's myths. The definition of a myth is, "A commonly believed but false idea," and the dieting and fitness industry is full of them. Myths come from an idea that a person or a group of people have, and whilst their intention is innocent, ideas catch on fast; and without any challenge or proof, people share it and market it, and it changes, sometimes changing the truth.

This once truth or experience even now serves a generalised concept. One example of this is, "Don't eat carbohydrates after 5pm if you need to lose weight." We can always find evidence for and against this type of statement, but for someone who struggles to lose weight, this has mileage through the desperation of trying to find anything at all that may help that individual. There is so much information, but very little is verified and accurate; and as a coach, I would prefer access to outside information to be limited, and instead let yourself be your own guide, from within. It is a very powerful way to live.

Your health cannot ever be controlled and legitimised by clever marketing tricks or a statement that lacks context and is being used generally without any sound basis. Remember, we will believe what we want to, because of our frame of reference—our beliefs are aligned that way.

I want you to look for your own answers from within first. Then, and only then, if you get to know yourself first, are you able to support yourself with outside information. Many people are in a stage of learning called unconscious incompetence; that is, they don't know that they don't know! To open that perspective and move them along, it takes an aware, wise, and gifted person, with good intentions.

I seek to get you out of your comfort zone with new information, because only then does true transformation for you happen. It has to be an integrated approach to change in mind, matter, and spirit. Your job is to learn and continue learning, become your own master, create your destiny, and live every day to your biggest potential.

Self-knowledge, awareness, and access to it are important when it comes to health. As you have read so far in my book, there is more against us in being healthy than any time before. Health today is controlled by money makers, and if we continue to sell our health to someone else, we will get stuck; because when we get caught up in a web of misinformation, they will have practically locked us in and thrown away the key.

Data can be manipulated; there are clinical trials sponsored by companies that invest in manipulating evidence only for their cause, so be wary of what evidence actually means, and where it is from. I love science, so evidence-based information will be something that I look at, but not all of it is truly independent. We have seen that with the fats and saturated fats in the diet, and decades of misinformation on this, giving rise to the convenience of low-fat processed food, it is very profitable to the food industry.

You can head over to www.JourneyIntoRealHealth.com to see the top common myths believed by people. You may be stuck in one or more of them, and that may actually be getting in your way to improving your health.

You decide for yourself what rules and boundaries you want to create to get you living a dream life with health as your foundation. Without it, I am afraid anything else you build for a happy life will be unstable and may collapse in an untimely manner.

Question for you:
"What beliefs do you have about health,
generally and specifically for you?"

Guiding principle:
"Information that is evidence based can be untruth; your inner guide and intellect can be exemplary if you only listen and use it."

The Food Industry

On one hand, we can now easily access food—all kinds of food. We all have too many food choices and ways of eating. This has caused so much confusion for people who literally don't know where they stand with food these days. My family shopping bill has always been expensive compared to some others mums of the same size family, because I have made a commitment to buying nutritionally rich foods, in organic vegetables and fruit, organic whole meats, and then minimally other things, like some organic dairy and grains. Many parents try really hard to provide the best for their children. I think there is this misperception that people don't know anything about good/bad food. We do, really we do, and although I think education about the functionality of food needs to be better, we all have a really good idea as to what foods we are meant to be eating. The danger is putting foods in good and bad groups, which if we set as a rule, can turn on a very powerful mechanism within ourselves through our self-talk, an internal dialogue of communication that can be very disruptive to our health and actions with what food we choose and why. I mention more of this later in this book.

So for those who have always eaten right, or eat right 80 percent of the time, why do they fall sick then? There is a huge campaign on nutrition being the saviour for everyone, but I think it is still damaging because it is based on the assumption that people don't know how to eat—they do! Food is not used for physiological reasons, like it is meant to be, but for emotional reasons, and nutritionists and the media can push shiny, diamond encrusted cabbage down people's throats, and still that person chooses sweets! I fear that this new adventure for nutrition just sets the tone to get onto a different train that will eventually pull up at the same place as people are in now! I have many nutritionist colleagues who are brilliant at what they do, but they all say the same thing. But they also suffered lifestyle illness and are professional enough to heed their own advice and eat well, but why are they sick then? The other dimension is that we have many really young people in their 20s and early 30s who claim they are healthy, and they certainly look it; and these people are aggressively on social media, so we can get swept into their views, but I imagine that their youth will contribute massively to their health anyway. I know when I was 20 years of age, I was at peak health without any effort at all, but it is how you maintain that over the evolving years and experiences in life that really matters. Those would be people that I want to be associated with. They have hidden gems, knowledge, and wisdom, and usually these are the people who don't market themselves aggressively.

But today, why is the good food we eat not doing what it would have done before, like perhaps in my younger days? Well, to answer that in a simplistic way, there is much more at play with our health than exercise and nutrition, like stress and irregular sleep patterns, emotional disturbances, imbalances of lifestyle, broken spirits and struggling minds, and decreasing mental health, amongst some things. For now, let's assume those elements are all good, and let's concentrate on food.

Industrialisation and technology, as well as strong links for imports and exports, make it easier to eat fruit and vegetables grown thousands of miles away, far away from source; and for us to see it in our supermarkets, they have to look nice for salability.

Fresh produce is sprayed with chemicals, and although there are many papers that support that this has a minimal or no effect on human health, there is very little done on investigating the long-term effects of these chemicals over a long period of time. Furthermore, the soil that grows such food is becoming depleted of nutrients because of over farming and demand of food globally. This affects our environmental microbiome, and if we were to buy and eat foods from a local source, we would benefit from this microbiome. Then we have the added problem that most of our fruit and vegetables are transported in cold storage for almost too long—some say one year, and some say two years. No matter what the number is, it is far removed from its source, and under conditions that are not best for maturity and optimal nutrition. It is more about getting these into supermarkets awaiting eager buyers that want to buy fruit and vegetables that look nice. So much produce is wasted that does not fit the supermarket standards and policies. The same food gets wrapped in plastic. We therefore think that by choosing fresh fruit, we are getting the nutrition we expect, but we don't.

Part of the mix of our weekly shopping can be processed foods, and if you look at the number of ingredients, I would be impressed if you even knew what they were! I know I don't always myself. Manufacturers don't have to tell us in entirety what they put in food. They can hide ingredients because they are so small in content, yet can be detrimental for us long term. If there are more than 4–5 ingredients, or any hidden processed sugars, then it gets put back. I have maintained cooking freshly made food. I even maintained that at university, and did not succumb to the dilemma of being a student hard pressed for cash to buy good food for themselves. I chose differently on how I spent my money with what I had coming in.

Budgeting was important, and I managed and developed a weekly menu for myself that was healthy, wholesome, balanced, and diverse, and took next to little time and money. That was a win.

It is not a hidden fact that processed foods are unhealthy, yet we see them flooded in food outlets. So many ignore or even dismiss this. Why? For those who are hard hit with cash, they consistently spend on drinking and cigarettes, but then they moan about how they can only afford a can of beans, and how hard done by they are. We can become victims of processed food, as they are addictive. Manufacturers invest a lot of time and money in taste forums, tweaking what most people like to taste, and most will play about with salt content and sugar content. Our brain quickly learns the "hits" it gets from food through sugars and artificial flavours, packaging, and the emotional connection. Further embedded in our minds is the copious brainwashing messages through advertisements. I don't see a single advert for fresh fruit and vegetables–only for processed junk!

Sadly, people do fall for this "hit," because it plays on their emotions; it fills gaps in people's lives, and it is so easy to see it and go buy it, without any self-interrupter that is wiser than the advert's call to action. There are many that are lobbying for more responsibility from food manufacturers, retailers, national government, and the public health department, to pay attention to advertising this way to us and to our children. I find that campaigning this way will help and is welcome, but it's a long shot. There are measures in place and behind the scenes—a network, an organised ring of people who are set to gain, and are gaining, at our cost. After all, they argue that it is "free will" and not enforcement that allows you the choices, and they are right! The choice of how we are in our health is unconditionally our own thing. It is 100% our responsibility. We gain greater power and momentum in this to change ourselves first. Don't wait for them. Make your own choices of what foods you eat, and start now.

If the demand of such processed foods falls through our buying choices, then it forces the food industry to supply us with better foods, like our fruit and vegetables, and to make them more accessible and cost effective. Perhaps they may go to a local producer and help local farmers. The price of food today challenges many families on low income, who genuinely want to be healthier and feed themselves and their children better food. Many food budgets are compromised for their annual holiday away together, so it's a difficult plate spinning exercise for many. The false perception is to buy discounted foods, which are usually processed stuff that are on for a good deal; but again, it's just a trick to get you to buy more of what you don't need. When you have excess at home, there is a compulsion to eat it, further fueling disease.

Think about the real cost to your health.

What is cheap now will cost you and everyone else more later.

It is a trap!

Work out what you really spend on food and drink, and be brutally honest with yourself. If you think like me, and 80 percent is on the good stuff weekly, then come join my tribe. If it's higher than that, then brilliant—I will join you! Once you have this worked out, you will be able to shift where you spend, and on what foods. Don't worry about what the kids will say. Yes, if they suddenly see a multibag of crisps missing from the cupboard, they will moan, and they will open all the cupboards because they think it's hidden. But when they can't find it, they will eventually forget about it and get over it. It's more likely that YOU will miss it more. Am I right?

I am not saying don't buy the crisps, but mindfully reduce these types of foods over a few months, and you will start seeing a saving.

So again, this change starts with you, your methods, and involvement with food in every area, from shopping to cooking and serving it, and then eating it enjoyably.

Another possible consequence is that we may see a re-emergence of local independent shops that have been decimated by big retailers and the 24-hour opening. They can't compete. The high street and local village landscape had 2–3 in every village, as well as local independent farmers' shops with fruit and vegetables straight from their farms, with produce stacked on themselves and not wrapped tightly in plastic. They provided something much more valuable in our food: good organic and nutritionally whole food that we are designed to eat.

My kids are incredibly mature in their decision processing; they are aware of their minds and what they say and speak. They have an amazing capacity to balance things and see things from different perspectives, and I have never had any problem with feeding them fruits and vegetables, like many parents complain about. However, from observing parents, I can see how this may play out in their homes. The interesting thing is that when the same children come to my home, they eat the vegetables and all the fruit, and they are relaxed and have such a great time with it. It's like they know how to access their innate desire for good food but in certain environments that give them permission to eat intuitively, and I guess I am very relaxed around food. I think that's it! Parents are too much in their head when it comes to mealtimes and what they should be getting their children to eat, and the focus is all wrong. Relax, and you will see a massive difference; you will understand this more when I talk about attention seeking traits later in this book.

The food culture of today is about convenience, and the whole and most natural experience with food and what it is, has become a chore. There is always something more important than eating in the Western culture. And let's face it, that is where most lifestyle diseases have taken root. Cooking is labelled as a chore, and if you can avoid it, then the motivation is going to be very strong. We can't blame the food manufacturers for that. We asked for it, and the food industry responded, to our detriment and their accomplishment, with ready meal markets, and cutting our vegetables and packing them in plastic so that they can quickly and easily be served up as a stir fry. They allowed for us to change our taste buds to accept more artificial, processed ingredients lacking in quality; but it is convenient, so that's okay, right? Seriously, if you don't like cutting some vegetables, get a processor or chopper, and if you don't have time to prepare a good meal, you need to look at what you are spending your time doing.

Most of us actually have a degree of a dysfunctional relationship to food, because food has become entertainment and part of creative art. I don't mind that, because it can still be that and healthy. But there first needs to be a will to do it. So many pay lip service to it and fail to integrate it seriously into their lives. They cannot manage their minds with it, and this is what is targeted when the food industry targets to your needs, vulnerabilities, and a weaker mind, with food and drink. If you ever shop when you are hungry, notice how much crap there is in your shopping trolley! I still remember the flake advert: a beautiful woman getting in her bath whilst biting her crumbly flake. It was very sensual and hit all the marks for pure pleasure and relaxation. Good food didn't need to be marketed back in the day, but now it does, to balance our perception of what food is, to educate us all, and to make it more appealing than processed food—maybe that's what food manufacturers can pay attention to. There are very few adverts with fruit and vegetables; if any, they are on processed, manufactured, packaged food. Why?

I love a flake, and it was my favourite bar of chocolate as a teenager, and I remember how many times I would watch the same advert, which was imprinted into my brain to go get it every time I was feeling peckish. Advertising on television is powerful and can influence us in decisions; we know that, so let's just not forget it—be mindful!

The industry watches for trends and then sets the wheels in motion as to how to get the end user buying.

We wanted low calorie foods that were also convenient, so that was set by the dieting industry that fed us that watching calories was very important for our weight management. We got and still have low-fat food, yet it is laden with sugar! People are obsessing about "fat" food, yet it is sugar—the refined stuff—that is the culprit to so many health problems. So now we don't want sugar anymore, so we have sugar alternatives that no one knows enough about, like artificial sweeteners and sugar derivatives, because it is important to get a product that tastes right that will get people buying more and more. They really do not have our health in mind, but sales and branding; and the sad truth is that some people know what's in their food and still buy it and eat it. It's always about sales and profits. Artificial sweeteners that are in so much of our foods that we eat, are now known to be controversial; in fact, many studies have proved that there is direct correlation for the increase in obesity around the world.

We need to stop blaming others for our own short sightedness, and start collaborating and sharing knowledge that has a positive impact for everyone. Yes, I would like complete transparency with all ingredients; in fact, they have recently changed the labelling into a traffic light system, from red, amber, and green, but we need to go further than that. We need to categorically state what is natural and what is unnatural in our foods. If we only bought whole food, then there would be no problem, but people are skirting around in aisles in supermarkets, buying preformed chicken for their kid's sandwiches. This is NOT chicken. It may taste bland and look the right colour, but touch it, and it's slimy and smells very processed. Top that with the bread that comes along with it in sandwiches, and your kid has just had one important ritualistic meal that is wholly processed. Is it any wonder they are so hungry when they come home, and they eat more crap, like crisps, chocolates, and sweets? Ask any shop near a school what they make in sales straight after school finishes!

Instead, I buy a whole organic chicken, oven bake it with beautiful Indian spices, and it's healthy and wholesome. My kids have a sandwich filled with that, or they make a salad for themselves. It also stretches to my lunch the next day. It is healthy and cost effective, and takes me no time at all—it's the oven that does the work, not me!

I don't want to be eating aspartame or fructose syrup added in for false taste and, even if it says it is not part of the ingredient list, it's in there; if they put the tiniest portion of it, they don't have to declare it on the packet. We have overcomplicated things collectively, and we are all to blame for the crisis that faces humans and nature today. It is the simple pleasure of food, relationships, and nature that we need to connect with again to simplify our health. I am convinced of it; and funnily enough, I have encouraged and practiced this from the beginning. In my culture and as an Indian, the wisdom of our ways is short of miraculous in its therapeutic teaching and ways with food, family culture, and so many other ways. However, the saddest thing is that whilst I am in the generation that values it, and understands it because of experience, it is dying fast as we approach the Western ways of doing things and eating. I have observed how South Asians here in the UK are sicker now than ever before; in fact, many younger generations don't have the same health as their grandparents still have. That is concerning, don't you think?

India today is wealthier and even more self-sufficient and high in spiritual guidance, but it is infiltrated with the Western diet and way of life, and the sum of its effect is that it is now leading in diabetic illness globally. If we could just stick to the diets that our bodies are used to culturally and traditionally, and not mix too many things up, then we may be able to correct illness back to health. South Indians in the UK are known to have their own traditional foods, but because they also now mix it up with doughnuts, loads of bread, sugar, and all the foods sold in the modern supermarket, that's what is causing problems for them. The diet is largely vegetarian, and the carbohydrate content is ridiculous, and then they wonder why they have problems with diabetes and linked diseases. It is well known that Indians who come into this country, from India or Africa, put on so much weight that their relatives back home do not recognise them. When they go back for a long summer holiday, they arrive back lighter because they ate foods that their bodies are used to—they have a unique microbiome that prefers those foods.

Yes, the quality of food is one thing, as I mentioned above, but more than that, it is the mix of traditional food with Western food that poses the biggest threat to their health. The mix just does not work, and they would be better sticking to the traditions of their food, which are passed on by knowledge from parents and grandparents and their grandparents.

Food is such today that we have to question it.

Question for you:
"What is it about your food and eating
that needs to change to give you better health?"

Guiding principle:
if you wait for the food industry and all that lobby for better food,
to get round to helping you, you will be waiting a long time. Why
wait? Be the change that you want."

Are We Just a Big Social Experiment?

Do you ever get the feeling that your life is just not your own? If you work for someone else, then that feeling may sometimes be intensified, and if you are an entrepreneur like me, I still get that feeling sometimes, because there is a lot we cannot always control or influence. It is like you have to be so thick skinned, and sometimes you feel unable to stick to what you know is right for you, and this can be a very lonely place for some time until you meet like-minded individuals that have the same awareness. The workings of the world are so disjointed and inaccessible. Change that is so needed in the world, is so slow and at times unsuccessful. You know that when it comes to your health, and our collective health, there is more wrong and against us that we have to battle through. The collusion between industry and governments are incredibly damaging for our collective health.

So much is based on far-outdated models—the way of the working world, the way our food comes into our lives, the way education has stripped away creativity and autonomy in our young, competition that breaks us apart rather than building us up, our fragmented society, outdated leadership models, the way we treat each other, the way our healthcare institutions make us sicker, and how illness rather than wellness is encouraged. Mankind faces disease on a massive scale, and our inaction and actions will be responsible for the demise of our precious planet. We all need to step up and take serious responsibility, and do our part for the greater good. Today, there is still time, but we need to act!

I am calling for more transparency with what we are encouraged to buy or spend time with. Companies need to be kept responsible for their staff, and every person that is with them, no matter what position they find themselves in. Companies need to invest in structural changes and areas where the wellbeing of their staff is protected and encouraged. I would like a health and wellness statement and implementation strategy for every individual company, including the SME market. Being small does not excuse the way you treat your staff, or yourself for that matter.

How well are we really educated to cook, understand the food we eat, and understand the need of nutrition and its functionality in our bodies? Someone, somewhere, decided to take away this part of the curriculum in our schools. They took away lunch time that lasted a little longer, to push more of the academic curriculum. Teachers are sick for long terms, and going part time, which means one subject is taught by two to three teachers who don't know what the other is doing, giving a disjointed experience. Teachers blame the governments, but they can choose to do their best with what they do have. I would prefer to home school rather than send them to teachers who lack passion and stay on the complaining frequency.

Many do not know how healthcare works today, or how they are labelled by doctors in order to deal with symptoms. Doctors cannot know everything, and frankly are not fully informed today. They are stuck in a bubble of theory, sometimes outdated, and then they don't have the time or the necessary resources to learn what they need. I remember the time when my second baby (my second daughter) was born, and a few weeks into her life, she started coughing, being unwell, and bleeding through her nose while having a temperature. Despite a few visits to my GP, who sort of said that I was a worrier and needed to "chill out a little," and that there was nothing wrong, a few hours later, we decided to take our girl to the A&E department because my intuition was more powerful as a mother than a doctor's opinion—he simply judged me, taking up less than 5 minutes of his time, when he could be seeing other patients. She had pneumonia, and her oxygen levels were very low; she was in hospital for two weeks and could have died. Is medicine at primary care now all about prescription distribution medicine? I think it has solved the symptom (plaster therapy) but ignored the cause, which is where real medical practice lies or should lie.

My doctor today, works for her money, because I challenge her when I need to. She likes it; it allows her grey matter to work. Otherwise, her job is so mundane as a GP, seeing mostly people with coughs and colds, and asking for magic cures when, in fact, symptoms like these are our bodies innate way of communicating to us to slow down to fix our own immunity. We are also to blame for this modality of our instant gratification culture that demands everything NOW.

Our bodies are much more knowledgeable. Medicine and drugs have a place; they have helped and are helping, but overprescribing or even inappropriate prescribing has cost us in more ways than we know or imagine. So, we also need to do our part with our physicians, and not demand treatment because we can't be bothered to sit still and trust our bodies to do the work that they were designed for, in terms of healing mostly minor ailments—give it a few days; don't instantly gratify yourself with our health service. If being seen cost you money, you would stop right there, would you not? If it was anything serious, then go, but I am talking about colds and flu, sore throats, and headaches.

There is this unconscious teaching that if something is offered for free, then it can be abused, and that it has no value and it is your right to abuse, and that goes for people that are working in our healthcare system, and also their customers. If not mindful, staff can be entrenched in a perception that if a customer is not paying for the service, then why should they be polite or even helpful. There is such a massive range of people in our healthcare service: ones that are beyond compassionate and kind, and those that treat you like a nobody. My patience and compassion have been tested many times with some NHS staff, as well as staff in education. There is so much inconsistency across the two platforms, and that's the problem. Archaic and rigid leadership is not appropriate in today's world. We need our healthcare and education staff to be happy, and that means being healthy and feeling fulfilled. Yes, they will face challenges like we all do, no matter what and who we are, but being healthy inside and out, in mind, body, and spirit, with purpose and fulfillment in life, turns those challenges into small obstacles that can be conquered. That will improve their level of customer service.

It is so common that people that live with some chronic illnesses are on multiple medications, so what evidence is there that these multiple medications work in synergy together. We know that the food we eat

76

can somehow interact adversely with some medications, but are people who take them told of that?

I have already touched on our obesogenic environment and the mixed messages from various sources. On one hand, they encourage us to stay healthy by eating well and exercising, and yet they approve very unhealthy food outlets to flood our streets. Our high streets are packed essentially with food, fashion, and banks. That's it. I have nothing against enterprise, but let's balance out our town centres so that they are healthier and more family friendly, and have social and public health at their heart. I want to see a different high street, with healthy, wholesome foods and drinks, spaces created for people for meditation and stillness, and drinking water that is accessible to all—something that is not recognised and is so undervalued for our health. We need the re-emergence of organic meat and fresh fruit and vegetable markets, and an expansion of this kind of main market into bigger towns and villages. It's instead disjointed, inconsistent, and missing genuine heart for people's lives. You get my point. It just makes getting healthier and staying healthier so much more difficult, and that, in my experience, is the number one reason why people do not embark on this journey. They can't do it on their own. It's too difficult, and they feel alone following a path that goes against the normal.

I have been on this journey and have taken many clients on it; and yes, it's hard, but it's incredibly liberating and powerful, and worth every challenge that is put in your way. What you will notice is that I point out that so much is wrong in our world, but I can't hack each system that needs changing for everyone's benefit on my own. I need you and those who are already like me, who have walked that path and are enlightened to the real problems that no one talks about because of the fear of challenge—the challenge to our food, education, government, politics, healthcare, and organisational systems that are making us ill.

With so much sewn up in such an organised and influential way, my question is, are we just a social experiment, infallible and expendable?

I see a future model where everyone gains, and where wealth and opportunity are shared rather than belonging to only a few.

What type of legacy do you want to live and leave? Death is inevitable, but that is not meant to get you to say, "Well, what the hell; I am going to die anyway, so I may as well enjoy myself," because that is not your purpose! You are meant to live your life responsibly, to learn something about yourself, and to live and leave something that is impactful on the rest of us so that we can pick it up and run with it, so that we can live longer and leave our legacy too—and so it continues, the meaning of life and death.

Our other higher needs are to be social creatures, happy and uncomplicated, to leave our egos behind, and just learn to entertain and be with each other; to stop overdoing or over-being every now and again, and use techniques like meditation and mindfulness exercises. Get a coach to keep you accountable to your dreams and purpose so that you can stop looking for answers from outside; learn instead to look inside. I have written an extra piece on "Choosing a Coach", head over to www.SanjayaPandit.com for that. If you need to lose weight because it is putting pressure on your heart, then lose weight. Why risk days thinking about losing weight? It may be too late. Health is about learning and understanding it as a priority, and the urgent nature with which it speaks. Get it resolved no matter what. Your heart will thank you for it, and if you have a good heart, you have everything!

Look at what you give your children, and see what has been packed in their school lunches that they regularly eat. Many parents complain that the good foods are not eaten, but the crisps and chocolates are, and they give them that because then that child at least is eating something. That is not even going to get better until you decide to stop feeling sorry or guilty, and brave up to include the foods that you would much rather they eat, and not pack their lunches with the distractive foods that are quick energy and calories but empty, and hence have no nutritional benefit whatsoever. What you give your young is what they become when they are adults, so your job as a parent is fundamental when it comes to healthy adults.

They may make a fuss, and may even throw the lunch out and not want anything, and make you feel so guilty, but stay grounded and don't get invited to a mind game that gives you emotions like guilt and fear. No child will go hungry to the point it overrules their survival, and it is at this point that they will be thankful for that chicken salad and raw vegetables you packed.!!

Preventative measures are smarter, active solutions.

Question for you:
"How can you trust yourself enough to know what is right for you?"

Guiding principle:
"Stop letting others screw with your health;
you are not their puppet."

Eating Quality Versus Quantity – The Correct Version

So we have ascertained that the convenience foods are not always of best quality. We simply don't know what is in our food, and sitting in plastic wrappers all day is far from the way it would be if it was growing and we picked it straight from a tree or dug it up from the earth. Convenience over quality, as we continue our busy work, family, and social schedules, comes at a cost to our health.

In the developed countries, it is a known fact that we are the most overfed and yet the most undernourished. It has become so industrialised with efficiencies for mass scale, that the natural goodness of our food has been depleted. There are too many loops that our food has to go through before it is even eaten by the consumer—you and I.

An added problem is that we have a "lack" mentality with food. The irony is that most of us have too much food, and it is accessible for 24 hours now, with UberEats and Deliveroo, and yet we spend most of our time in a mindset of lack when it comes to food, so we tend to overeat. We try to be too clever for our own good, by eating every bit worth the cost of what we have bought it for, and that is a "lack" mentality in progression. We need to break away from ritualistic eating, as I call it, and to get away from the mindset that we need quantity (big portions) to be full! This old belief, dictating that you can eat until full, is unhelpful, and although each of us has a different threshold to this, it is important to note exactly this: We are all different. Our stomachs can distend until sometimes painful, before we stop; and then for some, they keep eating beyond the pain.

How much is too much depends on your size and threshold for discomfort and, of course, what your mind is saying at the time of eating. We must get into eating only when we physically require it, rather than the old-fashioned conditioning of breakfast, lunch, and dinner. Also, we need much smaller portions than we all currently have. Having a huge meal in one sitting is not the best for digestion either. We just need enough, that's all, to keep our metabolism going; and yes, I know, what's enough for some?

I know how difficult this is to break out of, because all of our work and education systems don't allow us to eat mindfully, or when we individually require it. Eating is followed around work and school rather than the other way round, because it is an inconvenient thing we all must do, and even when there are lunch breaks, people don't always follow them appropriately or seriously. Some people, however, in organisations, graze all day and every day, and some miss important food breaks to refuel themselves, and keep going on empty. These are extremes contributing to people's ill health and the growing obesity crisis we are seeing. Our education system (our young) mirrors organisation's working practices (our young future selves), so by the time you start working, it is ingrained in us that our employer, and time we give there, is more important than our functional need to eat well and hydrate. So it is time to look at your own eating patterns. What influences it? How often do you ignore feeling hungry or thirsty; and then what do you do? And with what?

What actually happens during your lunch break? It is worrying that people will miss meals or dismiss genuine physical hunger signs for what they call more important stuff. Could your car run on empty? By missing meals or eating inappropriately, you will naturally be ebbing toward more urgent hunger, and more than likely, when you can finally get away from the mindset of work, you will suddenly remember how hungry you actually are. But because it really cannot wait, it is easier to pick up something unhealthy to deal with the cravings.

Many people overeat in the evening, after work, to make up for the lack during the day, and if you are not very active in the evening, and slumber in front of the television or the settee, then that is again not helpful to you long term. You will have problems. It is the same again for children who come back from school; they overeat if they are allowed. Do you see how the behaviour of young people in school mirrors the working adult population? Your body is not designed to work that way, so you have to help it. Most people eat vast amounts of food after work to make up for not being able to eat during the day. Even if you don't gain weight, this practice is detrimental, and you may find there are clues in other aspects of your health, like how you sleep, inflammatory conditions, heartburn, tiredness, and headaches, to name a few. You may not have any signs, but you are not immune; changes go on deep inside you, and you may simply not know.

Always pick quality over quantity with food. Small amounts of quality ingredients in your food will last you until your next meal. Just ask people who focus on this as a part of their daily lives, how awake and productive they are, and how their quality of life actually improves through such simple basics. Making sure we have quality over quantity dictates a certain amount of preparation and thinking beforehand; without this, you are left at the mercy of what you can get from the shop or from your work canteen or vending machine. Perhaps someone has been kind enough to bring sandwiches and biscuits, and crisps and fizzy drinks, into your place of work, on a trolley, feeding the desire of the child within you to have a treat. You may only spend £3.20 for this, but what's the real cost? Every now and again, it's fine, like most things, but you have to become mindful of what nutrition you are getting for your money. Lunch boxes that kids have always contain sandwiches, crisps, and chocolate bars, and maybe a piece of fruit. Where are the vegetables? That meal contains processed bread, processed meat or cheese, unhealthy fats, and a piece of fruit—wow, sugar to add to the rest. Is it any wonder that children are famished when they come home, and how their concentration and mood deteriorates throughout the day?

The message is, eat quality and do not compromise. Quality is very affordable, and if we could just stop buying all the rubbish out there on a regular basis, then we would all save so much money, which could be used toward our healthier lifestyle or a reward for our good work—perhaps a small break away, or a spa day out, or a trip to the zoo with your kids.

Another point that is important to make is that we need to get better at understanding food labelling, because there is so much confusion in terms of what we need to be looking out for. The easiest thing would be to buy fresh fruit, vegetables, and meat, along with dried pulses, lentils, nuts, and seeds—with these foods, there is no need to even label them.

Think about it: food in metal or plastic containers, sitting on the shelf at a small price—how can that be good for us? Even frozen, from the list above, is better than processed foods.

How have we become so addicted to unhealthy foods? Let's get organised and plan our food from fresh ingredients, from a good variety, and those that really help our bodies to do what they are designed to do.

So, the solution is to prepare your food beforehand, and actually spend some time thinking about what you want to eat. I mean, we plan and prepare for every other eventuality in our lives, so why would you be missing this? It is no longer a viable excuse to tell me that you have not had time to eat at lunch because there was no time to get food, or that the right food was not available. No excuse, sorry. You had last night to prepare yourself a salad or a healthy pack up. You see, the thing that is at the core of this problem is not the food we choose but the time we allocate to thinking about and preparing the food we need to be eating. We are lazy, but we have time. Perhaps get off your phone for an hour—there, now you have time, right?

Empower your children to make their own things so that you are not having to make everyone's lunches, including your own—I can see why that can become a chore!

Seriously, make time and eat quality; and if you do, you will not need quantity, and your whole being will thank you for it.

Question for you:
"How can you eat better?"

Guiding principle:
"Ditch the crap—seriously, don't buy it; you will save money,
and your health will be better for it.
Instead, relearn to eat quality foods in moderation."

Mixed Messages

This is a big issue for many: managing your thoughts under the influence of mixed messages from a variety of sources and thoughts, and therefore the outcomes or actions that come about as a result of these thoughts.

You see, before you can get clarity into what health means to you, you have to find out what self- care messages have been working you— yes, **working you!** There is a reason I am confident and feel verified in writing this book; I have lived through every bit of it and have come out the other side, with loads of hard learning, which is what I am going to save you, to any degree I can. I cannot action the teaching for you, but I will continue to action it for myself, with you.

The power of influence does affect us, so if there are mixed messages within your own family, then that can be really hard to navigate. You know that saying that came out of your parents' mouths, which as a child you never agreed with, or just did not get? Except now you are just that, and almost robotically being influenced or saying it to your children? That's an imprint, and it's in your subconscious, which is driving those words and behaviours that were once frowned upon. They surface when we least expect them, and it can shock us. My children have regularly pointed out how I am like my own mum. Now, she is not all bad, but she, like many, has had mixed messages about things, but she does not realise it because she battles with her self-talk, those voices that give her confusion and contradictions. We love her, and it's not about blame but about educating yourself and knowing how you want to drive your life forward. Your brain keeps it stored, just like mine did, without realising.

It can be authoritative, dictatorial, critical, nurturing, loving, or liberating, depending on what part of the self it came from. These types of messages can be good or bad, but we rarely even notice the good ones. The bad ones, we notice, because it shocks us and wakes us up, just like a slap on the backside. So become more aware of what messages you give your health, and for those around you.

But imagine that you were put on a diet at 15 years old, just like Teresa, one of my life coaching clients, because of concerns with health or friendships at school. You felt and witnessed the concern of your parents. They tried so hard to fix it and ended up resorting to varying measures to get you to lose weight. You may have perceived this as not being loved for who and what you were, although you deserved to be loved no matter what you looked like or what size you were. Eventually, your difficult experiences of dieting made you swear that you would not put your children through it in any way. Then you find yourself doing just that—conditioning and influence at its best, but in the most unhelpful way. Sometimes our automatic thoughts and beliefs need an active force and energy to work against them. What we try to run away from gets closer. What you resist, persists.

Notice just how much time you spend with certain types of people around you, at work, at home, and in your circle of friends. You may really like someone overall but don't always agree with what they say or how they are. You may be too afraid to speak, and may even detach a little from them for fear of losing them all together. Either way, for the right or wrong reasons, I understand the difficulty.

It doesn't need to come to that. All you have to do is be alert on what influences you and if it is aligned to the way you want to live. It is about your priorities and values, and living by that in a helpful, healthy way.

Don't worry about people moaning or even gossiping. If they do, so what?! If they are critical, then don't expect them to take your view of the challenge or difference lightly. They may stop you in your tracks; let them. So what? You carry on. You may inspire a positive change in them as a result. If you have friends and colleagues who challenge your boundaries for better and more progressive self- care, then ask yourself if their influence keeps you stuck, and whether it takes you nearer or further from your goals. Equally, someone's challenge could be good feedback for you to get to your goals even faster, or drive your desire even more. Remember, there is good in everything, so just ask yourself whether they are going to take you nearer to your health desires and goals, or further away.

If you want to change something about yourself for the better, it can be uncomfortable, but that's okay; really it is.

Sometimes what comes up is not always expected, so any change can throw up all sorts of surprises, and you are going to have to deal with them head on. Remember, do not compromise your values. That will hurt you in the long term, and damage so much more than you are aware of at this stage.

Sometimes, with any change, it can feel overwhelming, and you can't see a way forward, and you can quickly feel that the best way is to go back where you came from, because looking back is less surprising— you know where that was, you lived it, and you are a master of your past.

This is due largely to your filtering system, beliefs, and experiences. So for you to take on anything from this book, you will either find you can resonate with some information, or for some, not so much. That's okay, because if you repeatedly read the bits that you cannot resonate with, it will make sense, and your awareness will be more open. Then make decisions from the open perspective.

Actually, I seek, and through this book, further seek to bring many points that make up a more holistic framework for total health for you, and because of the many layers it has, I do not expect everything to be implemented overnight. I can only hope that some work for you. That's a great start. Just make a start wherever you are in life right now!

Change that is meaningful takes time, but change for the better needs a first step; and by reading this book and fully understanding its true desire for you, that's your first step.

The points and information given throughout the book, that you find a challenge to relate to, may be an area for further learning and growth, so it is worth considering reading that part again. To gain health from a place you don't have, it is complex but worthwhile. This book gives a basic blueprint and a refreshing look at health from a bigger place rather than a precise script. There is enough of that around, and it cannot be rigid. I seek to create a solid foundation from which to build, and you are the most important change maker in this.

I know that different aspects of health are so fragmented, and my mission is to make it whole—join the dots, so to speak—and then use an implementation strategy that will help you get and live healthy wherever you are. The foundation of health as a whole has never been taught this way, because people within the health sector have to market themselves in one thing; and that's what they are taught by business consultants. Attaining health is not a business, but your health is absolutely *your* business. I think we can do better. With health, it has to be the whole offer; otherwise, it just becomes a home improvement project. You know, the DIY jobs that need doing, and you start on one, and when that one is finished, you move onto another, and what you find is that the first job you started with needs doing again, and it never ends—it's like a never-ending cycle. For so many people, that's their experience of health, because they are trying to avoid death and illness, but if they decided to shift their paradigm into living well and with health, then it may not be so tough, and things just conspire to help you live just like that. Balancing life does not have to be so punishing. Home improvements are projects within projects. The wear and tear of the environment we live in and use is far higher than the wear and tear on our bodies, because our bodies are living beings, and with life comes restorative recycling.

It is there to serve you.

Are you serving it?

You are your best friend, and if not, then work on yourself to be just that. Treat yourself well, with purpose and meaning. Health transcends the whole of you, and it is when the focus is on the whole of you that a beautiful picture evolves that seeks to complement your inner and outer world, in harmony. We don't get taught this ever. Can you imagine our children knowing this and teaching this to their children, and how our world would change?

The more we comply with technology, the way the world is now, the further we disconnect from our health. For some, it's just too late, and for others, the impact of disease shows that they have been disconnected somewhere, and influenced in ways that have been unhelpful. There is time to rest and restore. Imagine that there are no limits to what you can experience; that is pure joy and abundance. That is how powerful the gift of health can be.

We try to cheat death, but death is inevitable. I think differently. I don't want to die because of ill health but because it's my time, and I am done and have played my tune. I won't cheat myself out of that. I have been born for something important. Dying at a good old age, having experienced a full and meaningful life with nothing wrong with me, is the thing I would hold dear; and when it's time, I will go gladly, but I don't want to be cheated. I will then gratefully surrender to my next phase. Will my life, after I expire, be celebrated? Not because I was a celebrity but because I had an impact in the world, from a place of humility and genuine intention without the privilege or elite background, that impacted both my world and yours! It acts as an imprint. I don't want people to have a premature death, or for people to lead a low quality of life, prolonged only by medications; but instead, I want to empower them to take the gift of health gratefully and respectfully.

There is much work to do, because we chase other commodities and do not give attention and intention to our health and lives before we get to that time, and now have to face no one but ourselves to answer difficult questions on what that was all about. It can leave you empty, guilty, and now seeking desperate answers, because death is now very real, and you understand that you haven't lived YOUR life—you start on your health journey way too late. That was never the intention when you were given the gift of your human life. You are, like each of us, responsible for your own wellness.

It does matter what other goals and achievements you intend to accomplish—making millions, taking over industries, being known as an expert in your field, having a home with a happy family life, or perhaps being destined to be the best employer, who is dedicated and committed to their company vision—but none of these attributes are possible when you lack whole health. There is nothing worse than making your money, only to find that you can't enjoy yourself. Illness is a big liability.

Building personal and business empires in your life, under rocky foundations, is a certainty for deep fault lines that will raise a tsunami of devastation.

Life can be unpredictable; your health, you can predict. From this place, any curve balls can be managed with confidence. It is a choice—your choice.

So start now; what does your self-care look and feel like? What messages have an influence on what you think and do? Messages are from parents, sisters, brothers, or teachers; in fact, anyone who had a significant influence on you at any time.

I remember messages such as having to eat everything on my plate, and then I would get told that I was putting on weight and needed to eat less. Yes, it's completely irrational and confusing. That confused state left me eating more, and finishing everything on my plate, even at the age of 35, and then wondering why I was putting on extra weight, because I could not understand myself and my ways. You see, the "finish everything on your plate" was profound for me, because it meant not wasting food that could easily go to poor people; so in fact, I treated myself as the human dustbin, but I was not really helping the poor with my guilt-induced feelings. I got fat, and they remained poor! Of course, once I became aware how ridiculous this was, I then stopped putting so much on my plate, and I could finish the right portion for me, which satisfied my hunger and made sure I concentrated on the quality of my food and not the portion size.

My self-care tactics to curb gaining any more weight was to stop eating at the exact time my brain sent me signals that I was starting to get full, even though there was favourite food left on my plate. That connection—messages between my brain (thoughts) and my body (signals)—was because of better self-awareness and kindness shown to my body, as well as learning to trust it. I listened to my body and took what it said to me, seriously and with respect. When my mind would influence my messages in the past, I would try to overrule this intelligence; I chose what to listen to: the outdated message or my body in the given moment. We all have a demon—a saboteur voice— that lives in our heads, so until you know your mind and get it to work for you, listen to your body. Slowly, as time goes by, and you become more alert and aware, you will notice another voice that has always been there for the greater good of you, but it was masked by more disrupting voices. The voice that cares for you and loves you is your friend and ally for good.

What saboteur stays silent when it feels threatened? Its way is to throw you off target, to displace you, disrupt you, and stop you, and it's like a shape shifter—it will try to show up anywhere, anytime—it's unpredictable. Self-development and learning are the foundation of self-care. And how many of us get lessons in this throughout life? Like me, I found self-development when things were going wrong for me.

I had to force it on myself. I want self-development to have a place even when things are well. That's why I chose coaching, and in particular Co-Active coaching. I am blessed.

We have this view that our health is not in our hands, and that if something goes wrong, we can go to a physician to get it fixed, right? So it's less of a priority; we don't talk, learn, or teach enough about health at all, ever. It's something that parents wish for their kids but very rarely keep the task ongoing. It's only until we wean babies off milk and onto solid foods, and then when that period is over, then it's about getting them to see their dentist and optician, but rarely do they spend time talking about a healthy lifestyle with their kids—something has to happen before it becomes important. We don't need to lecture children if we, as parents, practice it and talk freely about what we are doing. Their observations are their learning. The worst thing a mum can do is not value herself and eat crap, and then expect her girls to be healthy and beautiful.

Not enough is talked about in terms of its benefits. We talk about careers and schooling for them, but we don't teach them; and without their health, it can all be for nothing. It's a lesser priority. It is when we finish work that we get time to go to the gym or walk or eat, if at all! It's when everything is sorted that we get "me" time.

I hope you have got the message that health is more than just being free of disease; in fact, WHO defines health in this way: "a state of complete physical, mental, and social wellbeing, and not merely the absence of disease or infirmity." And I would go a little further and include spiritual and emotional health. The whole thing is integral to our daily lives and must be weaved into the fabric of our days, from as early as we can get it to be, and that means teaching everyone we love to do the same. They can find different ways, and there is flexibility to own it their way, but there are some basic and core principles I allude to in this book that cannot be negotiated.

We can renegotiate time spent on other things, even for five minutes for a quick walk, a healthy snack to energise our bodies, a power nap without guilt, or stopping and sitting quietly so that we can enjoy a moment of peace and serenity, and work on our internal bodies and spirits, and connect to our hearts. Once health is established in all these areas in a balanced way, you will think, work, and feel amazing. There are no mixed messages here. If you feel guilty in doing this, then you need to look at what messages (thoughts) are creating that feeling in you.

Your job is to keep this awareness going on your mixed messages (thoughts, feelings, and behaviours), and especially those incongruent thoughts and actions. Working on the three elements is like having three very close and intimate friends, who depend on each other and have a contribution to one another to create a sum that is way more powerful than its individual parts.

Please go to my bonus page to download a template to work with at www.JourneyIntoRealHealth.com

Question for you:
"What are you becoming aware of
when it comes to mixed messages on health?"

Guiding principle:
"Become aware of the outdated and incongruent messages
to your health; be alert, think, feel, and behave in a way
that is congruent with your best health."

Chapter principle:
"There is no doubt that there is a lack of truthful and consistent information. A lot about health relies on government advice and their allies to keep you confused and misinformed, and to give you mixed messages whilst keeping you in the past.
One day, fats are okay, and then the next, they're not. Well, which is it? Trends are tied up with misleading information, so qualify your information and research. If it's too good to be true, don't fall for it. Always use your intellect."

Chapter 3
The Challenges From Within You

It's Not Your Fault

Attaining health and protecting it is such an individual experience. You know this. You can learn to adopt good and necessary ways for yourself as long as you are truthful about it. I have worked with people who thought that pretending to make the changes whilst clearly not, was a smart thing. Health for some is about lip service; but without the serious action and implementation, it will fail. It seems to be the thing that people struggle with. This is partly due to people's motivation these days. Healthcare, and especially how to fix it, in all of its viewpoints, is big business, but it has become confusing.

My aim is to simplify health that once was, to allow people to seek updated and true knowledge, and to go back to basics and build again from there.

I know that a lot of what life throws at us can directly impact our health, but if you can respond to it with love, simplicity, balance, and gratitude, you can quickly gain composure, and things can be far better. At the beginning of any change that is meaningful to you, it needs your commitment and focus, and soon enough, you start to experience the fun and ease that shapes the change that you are on, naturally. Both life and health go hand in hand, and unless you are alive from within, you cannot truly live and show up authentically and bravely.

Many now agree that individualism, creativity, and being daring is pulled right out of us, during our entire school years, stressful parenting years, and through our working adult lives. I have witnessed unnecessary stress on children from parents, which they themselves had experienced through pressure from their parents, in order to attain success. It is not good enough to trade academics for creativity and individuality, and impress other's agendas on a young mind. Otherwise, what develops is an individual, or a group of individuals, who are very unsure of themselves but fit into a clone of puppets where strings are pulled by someone else, sometimes for their entire life. They may have a superb life in terms of material wealth and great success in their career, but their happiness is not always genuine.

What shows up eventually is the dormant force of a broken spirit, lack of individualism, and even lack of self-respect; and instead, anger and resentment. A life lived on someone else's terms is not a life fulfilled. Luckily, there are people who have been lucky enough to access both academics and creativity, and there are many like these who do an immense amount of good in the world—our change makers, for whom I have an immense amount of respect and gratitude. Here, you have the same opportunity.

If the value of health and wellbeing gets integrated into daily living, it sets a certain tone, and a space so that each and every one of us can define what we want within the framework, which takes into account what we each want for our health individually and then for the greater good of someone else.

Maybe someone likes cricket instead of football as a way of physical exercise, and we need to learn to not judge or feel offended if our thing has no take up. It's not about enforcing anything; the minute that happens, it becomes a rule, and we know how people like to break rules if they don't want it in the first place. It can push them so far that they show rebellion in a way that is unhelpful, and there is a risk of losing their motivation for health altogether.

Health only gets seen to if we have ill health, and then we try to avoid getting worse rather than starting from a point of proactivity. Let's ask how we can live to embrace health and wellbeing every day, in a preventative way.

Today, we try to enforce too many obligations with our health, which feel enforced and not through correctly thought-out choices: I must eat well; I must exercise this many times a week; I must lose weight; I must carry on smiling when I want to cry and hide. When they can't do it, they eventually switch off. There are some that are incredibly resilient and keep going even though the results are not coming in, and even they switch off eventually, having wasted so much money and precious time. How can that then work?

Sometimes a little help can help you go the distance with the results you desire. I run workshops that will help create plans so that you can own it, implement it, and take full responsibility for moving you from initial motivation to full blown empowerment.

I let the whole vision of health and wellbeing be part of my life and that of my family, and they get to pick and choose to make it their own. So we have some that sample different healthy foods to make them staples, and some of us do exercise in different ways, but we all exercise and we have different ways of relaxing. When I explain that to some families, their first thought is that it must be chaos doing different things, because they see only one way in their family. Yes, it takes some time to harmonise, but if the intention is set, and the ground work is done correctly, each of us can find a way to respect our similarities and differences, and connect with each other that way. I am sick of the one-rule-fits-all approach. That's the hidden need to control. It is interesting as to what can be behind that. We see that control aspect in outdated leadership styles at work and in institutions, and with parents, as well as with teachers in schools. I want change here as well.

Let individuals engage and submerge themselves into the overall vision and benefits. We all have the capacity of working things out for ourselves, but some information resonates more with some than others, and we can still have the value of health and wellbeing instilled in us all from the beginning. It's a collective vision and space with good enough flexibility for choice.

Sometimes you may recall that your life did not seem your own; instead, you were a mere vehicle delivering unresolved life experiences from parents or teachers—or anyone that was older that had not quite lived the way they wanted to in their life—and now that you had come along, it was a way of reconnecting themselves to the things they dreamt of for themselves. It happens a lot when people become parents, and it takes a huge amount of awareness to not have that automatically instilled into young minds. One important question to disrupt this is to ask, "Are you living your parents' dreams?"

There is nothing wrong with that except when you become aware that it is not what you want! And when you become aware of it, then you are torn between the past and the future, and what and who you really are. It is uncomfortable. Why would you not believe what your parents tell you? You believed them about Father Christmas and the Tooth Fairy, right? So if they tell you things outright, you perceive the messages that it doesn't matter about your health: "Eat right up until you are full; we are big because we are all big-boned in the family; just stay slim until you find a husband, and then he can look after you!" Some messages are bizarre, and they are linked to cultures of course, but the words spoken or the intent sent can get internalised, and then you are under that influence—it's very powerful.

Imagine if these messages were helpful and empowering instead of critical or unhelpfully nurturing, because it works both ways. There are all sorts of messages, and some culturally and environmentally defined. Being aware of all the outdated beliefs and thoughts, and habits and behaviours is a good thing because you are then in a position to change them with what is a better: more current beliefs, like health matters every single day of our lives!

Write down what you have been influenced with, what gets in your way, and how you may use those same beliefs to get in other people's ways? For example, "We will never be rich; we are not made for business."

Getting out of the way is essential in service of the person that you have with you, remembering that it's their life, they oversee their decisions and choices, and they can drive their own autonomy and focus that they need to experience in their life. Give them the responsibility of creating what they want for themselves. That way, they become their own masters and leaders.

Getting out the way is also to give them space for freedom, creative thinking, and a non-judgemental attitude. It is a small and valid technique that will go far to build the character of the person. They can then express themselves with confidence and assertion, and be authentic. We can therefore stop micro-managing them and allow them to learn key skills in managing their own life, putting it into free flow and ease, and equipping them with key skills to deal with any of life's challenges.

By the way, when I talk about the person, I am also referring to your own self-talk, which can express itself and stand in your way. Allow yourself to create from within. I share a coaching technique here, and that is to hold space for yourself and other people. You are not attached to your agenda; the space is only to process, create, and live freely with choices and open perspectives. Be present in the moment.

Allowing yourself and others a wide range of experiences, gives us all clarity into what we truly and deeply want for ourselves, and only then can we take full responsibility for our lives and live them to our fullest potential.

The challenges in health that face us today can be dealt with once you work from the inside out.

Question for you:
"What about your life is on the right path, where you feel authentic, fired up, and where it is easy and full of joy?"

Guiding principle:
"Wherever you are, whatever you are, is fine; accept it with all your heart and, from this place, create your master plan."

Peer Pressure Around You

Human beings are meant to thrive in community, so we are designed to be part of a pack. This allows for socialisation and for us to influence each other, and share knowledge, wisdom, and love. It also allows for us to be held in a safe space to explore what is necessary at any age. It is especially vital in younger years when creativity is natural and untampered, and we use it instinctively to find our way. We tend to take our lead from elders or the wiser ones. However, our world today very rarely respects our elders for wisdom, and there is a lot of disrespect for parents, whether together or apart through separation, divorce, and then re-marriage. We sadly tend to regard them as outdated and a pain or being in the way, nagging us into their old ways, although this does vary in cultures.

You only have to ask the elders in your community how they feel about the younger generation, if they have the courage to show their true feelings and vulnerability. This, in my opinion, is both sad and the sign of the times we live in, which is all me, me, me! We all need to embrace age and our elders being incredibly valuable to us all. The good thing is that they are with us far longer than before, and their wisdom is becoming an untapped goldmine, so encouraging them to stay healthy and whole for as long as possible would be an incredible thing. For them, it would be a wonderful way of living with extended purpose if they could feel included. In my culture, we are taught to have respect for our elders and our parents, and to hunger after the knowledge and wisdom they can share for our own wellbeing. Many have the formula for living well. Just ask the many centennials across our globe!

Our elders are more than babysitters or someone to go to for treats, biscuits, and cakes.

Living in fragmented societies does not allow for greater guidance, as we look to others for guidance and influence to further nurture our need for connection and belonging. We start to seek to survive and thrive through developing relationships and friendships at work, friendships from the outside, online, and in other ways. This is all good, and lots of good can come from it, as long as there is a balance and integrated variety. I know many people who have disrupted families, and they can become very close to another family or set of friends. I also know people who cannot find true friends anymore, and they go about life in a very lonely manner; worse still, pretending they have everything they need for a social life. We can also take on false relationships that are superficial and are accessories rather than having a mutual desire of deepening intimacy.

Whatever the situation, it is important that we share information and wisdom that comes from the heart and is true and genuine. As a scientific person, I love verification and science-based evidence, but as a coach, the wisdom and the verification that comes from within, having lived through experiences, far surpasses anything done in a laboratory.

It is not always possible to avoid being friends or being married to someone who doesn't want the best for you, even though they may not entirely know what their unresolved issues or agenda of sabotage is. It is impossible to know someone so fully, even though many couples think that they do. Life is constantly evolving, and to keep things together, you have to evolve as well. Peer pressure with certain subject areas like health, can be sabotaged in fear of changes to the relationships. What I ask people, regularly, who think they know everything, when there is no evidence of any knowledge about themselves—their blind self and unknown self—is, "How can you know someone when you don't know your deeper self?" If you want deeper and more meaningful, cherished relationships, start to get know yourself first.

Whilst many good things get shared this way, we have to watch for the not-so-good part of you, which comes from people who are the naysayers—the saboteurs, the witch (can be a man, a woman, or a child)—who magically entice you to be influenced in their ways. Do people like this even exist, I hear you ask? Yes, they do, so fish them out. I guarantee you have some.

Yes, and it's really hard to comprehend that people can be cruel and do not want the best for them or you, and that they are ridden with jealousy or are uncomfortable with your big dreams and desires, just because they are too smallminded to even begin to dream. We can literally take on other people's outdated beliefs and make them our own, without knowing what they influence in us. It's a very clever way of brainwashing. The worst is when they act so sweet and innocent; but gosh, when you truly expose them, you see red devils with horns, and harmful aliens, ready to watch you fall or take a wrong step, or distract you so that you can't even get started in anything you want. You will meet so many in your journey to optimal health. It may even be you doing that to yourself. For people, at least you know those that have an opinion about your health when you decide to correct it, but they stay really quiet when you are coughing your guts out because your lungs are compromised. Let's face it, they may even serve you a tray of cigarettes because they feel sorry for you, or a tray of cakes when they know you are trying to lose weight!

Mostly, you will be reassured to know that these "red devils with horns," and their behaviours and their words, come from a place of utter ignorance and lack of self-awareness for themselves, or for you for that matter. So relax; there is a solution. For now, just identify them, especially the ones in your inner circles without any blame or persecution. Your new awareness will be of service to them too, and I ask you to act with compassion and mercy to their ignorance. They do not know that they don't know.

In the meantime, watch out when you understand that you may not think of yourself as a natural leader, and instead prefer to follow someone else and be drawn into wrongful influence and peer pressure, especially if you are feeling vulnerable, which from time to time is normal. But they know that time, and they will pounce on you to get their way, ideals, and agenda.

We know quite clearly when we are in the company of something or someone that doesn't feel right, for reasons not entirely clear, but we stay with them in the hope that it will turn out okay—and does it? This false connection is what gets people hooked and addicted to social media groups, terrorism, false and inauthentic religious movements, and toxic friendships. What they then influence on us can be very damaging, as we all know.

It is a known fact that children growing up have always been influenced by peer groups, some good and some not so good. It is a matter of cultivating good tribes of people with and around you. The ideal would be a good balance of people who have similarities and differences, and with mutual respect. All too often, we feel that similarities are all that matters and what we need to focus on, and for a short time, that works; but it is so important to gain different perspectives and to learn from respected people. It is easy to go for people that are perceived as not being a threat or a challenge. People are actually scared of strength and passion. They go for what fits— what's comfortable. I hope that's not you. Who is the one person that challenges you for your own growth?

We need to belong to people that have the same or similar value-based living, and that is what exists in healthy families and healthy friendships. You can trust the information, knowledge, and wisdom shared here. It is also then vital to open the circle with different values, to work your appreciation, inclusion, and acceptance muscles. These are attributes that make a person whole.

Our sense of the world comes through communication with each other. We have sensors and radars, and we use collective information with collective knowledge to face challenges and aspire each other to greater experiences of our life. We influence each other in ways not always in our conscious awareness, and it is somewhat set in complex patterns. More importantly, once we are aware of it, we can learn from and make choices that are more about what and who we are, rather than what other people think of us.

The power of influence from peers is powerful. Imagine that it is there to serve our highest purpose and the best in us, and how important it is to be with people that are right for you. Imagine powerful, positive, authentic groups of people that can influence and listen well to each other without judgement. Imagine being part of that community every day.

Connection needs to be an easy flow, and one that builds each other up and shows a deep sincere understanding of each other. This is called intimacy. If intimacy is built correctly, then within it, there is a necessary place and purpose to challenge one another for the best in each other. Instead, how many friendships and relationships are only built on "when the going is good, it's good, but when it's bad, it's bad," and then there is no way an appropriate challenge can be raised— that's uncomfortable and scary. That's not the relationship I am after with people, because there is always a time when things become uncomfortable and need to be dealt with—do you think that is done well with someone that has a space for intimacy, or with someone that is superficial?

Now, let me further qualify what I mean by intimacy, because if you are happily married or part of a couple, have siblings or have parents, you may think that they are already qualified to be in this space, but that's not what I mean. Intimacy is not a given just by the designated role in relationships. It is a deeper authentic space for understanding, acceptance, and challenge, from the heart and not from ego.

I mean, how hard is it to tell someone, whom you know really well, that they are putting on weight, or that they need to lose some weight, in fear of being disliked, or afraid of their reactions and emotions? This is not intimacy, because the relationship is built somewhat on fear or disapproval. If you can, then that is the measure of your openness and true intimacy. Part of the reason that we can't improve other people's health is because we are too afraid to say anything to them.

You see, any ill health, and in particular chronic ill health, is slowly killing you. Are you prepared to have relationships with people that don't have the courage or voice to raise their concern and encourage you to do something before it's too late? No one likes the truth, but it's needed sometimes to save you. We would expect that in our partners, but even then, this does not happen quickly enough. We have gotten used to the soft-spoken approach, but it's a waste! Instead, I say to get it out, name it, be bold, and free people from their denial—the clock won't wait.

When we get influenced by peers who take us away from the direction and path that is best and true for us, it can open us up to sabotage, either directly from them or from their influence on our own internal voices, which can and does result in self-limitations. We listen to the internal voices that characterise someone else's original beliefs and what we action as a result. This may not be congruent to our own unique goals and aspirations. Think about it; there may have been a number of times you have witnessed or have personally experienced someone close to you sabotaging your dreams and ambitions, and how that influenced you to change your passions to a different direction. Or you stood still and forgot about what you were once so passionate about, and you put it on the back burner whilst watching them get on with their lives. Or perhaps it is you that has been the voice of sabotage in your peer group.

We have seen and heard how success can be sabotaged by someone in your peer group who believes for some reason that you will not succeed, and that the road or path to follow is crippled with challenges and difficulties. They may not out rightly say no, but they start to play with your mind, which was once clear but has now become a little confused. What were your dreams, in full glory? How much of those dreams were sabotaged? Well, perhaps it's time to clear what buries them, and bring them back to life. Let your dream breathe and see the sunlight, and let it be watered and nourished in order to grow again.

So, what is sabotage? Remember, it can be one person or a committee of them; it is a collective power force of doom and gloom and irrational opinions, not at all justified in what they are saying. Some people call it jealousy, but it's more than that when you look at it, like I have carefully. It starts with an awareness that they are being negative, and they are voicing their experience, or lack of experience, as their narrow frame of reference. We have a choice to listen to this and become influenced, or to continue on the path that we know is right for us despite objections.

So, I urge you to make a start today by taking a look at the timeline of things you wanted for yourself. Think on the times when peers were positive, who they were and are, and reconnect with them in a wholesome, grateful way. Who do you have in your sphere of influence that wholeheartedly supports you, and you them, and encourages you to live your life to its fullest potential? Who allows you to have a go at new things, without judgement and criticism, and to indeed bring something back from the past—that one distant and forgotten dream of a way of life or relationship, which you want again, and to manifest now? You know the difference between truly feeling alive with hope and ambition, and the corresponding energy and flow that comes with it. You also know the feeling of dissonance—a dead, hopeless feeling, monotonous in vibration—in fact, you can be around people that suck the life out of you. There are choices here! You can make the ones that make you feel alive and energised.

Do what you need to do, and move away; let them know why you are doing that, and then let it be. Let them process it, and if they truly have love for you underneath those layers of fear of something, then they will realise and connect to you in a better and more life-giving way. You deserve better, and so do they. It is through our fearless actions and boldness that we actually move the others from their slow death of unawareness and ignorance.

There is no need to shout or get upset at them when you realise that they sabotage you; so, show love and kindness and tolerance by asking them to allow you to give them feedback, and don't be afraid. If things break down after this, they were already broken, and you have not lost anything; instead, you have gained tremendous freedom. The feeling in you will become as light as a feather.

Question for you:
"When was the last time you looked at
the people you keep company with?"

Guiding principle:
"The company of people you keep is paramount to
your overall health. Let go of toxic people, or even the ones that
disguise themselves as sweet but wear a mask of a saboteur—
you know who they are, and have always known,
without listening to your inner guide."

Rebellion Within You – The Unhelpful Part

Can you think of a time when you noticed rebellion in yourself or in anyone else? Perhaps if you are a parent, you will be seeing this trait or behaviour in your children as they grow up. It is very normal in the teenage years, of course, and most people have experienced it through others or within themselves. What were you rebelling against? Did you want to break rules, risk things, and go against the status quo? Can you connect with how that felt for you and how it felt when you were caught in it? What was the impact on you from a rebellious acquaintance?

Or have you always been compliant—a "yes" person?

Rebellion and compliance are polar opposites, and the interesting thing is that they are functional states of thinking, feeling, and behaving from an overall childlike state. In transactional work, Eric Berne called it the child ego state. This ego state is a communication forum that you would experience when you display childlike thoughts, patterns, and actions. From here, you can understand how rebellion and compliance can serve or not serve. Rebellion has active energy (you can feel pumped up) to it, whilst a compliant state in this childlike ego, is one of submission with passive energy, to put it crudely. These ego states are with us for our entire lives. So you could be an adult in age but sometimes act like a child. Being rebellious can also be good if you can channel it the right way, or it can be chaotic and very unhelpful.

Let's look at it when it can be very unhelpful.

When we look at rebellion from a health perspective, we can see that it can be damaging and also really useful. However, knowing when and what you play out is key for the outcome. As we are in the chapter titled "The Challenges from within You," I want to focus on rebellious behaviours and thoughts that are a challenge to your goals in health.

You will notice that little children are really good at saying NO, and are not in any way bothered about it. In fact, they categorically think that being naughty not only gets them attention, but being naughty sets them off in giggles and cheek. Let's face it, children will push boundaries and test you, and they do it in a way that is innocent. Or is it?

To children, this time of rebellion could be a way of stating their points, being more visible, and working out how they need to experience the world around them. It is a time to challenge and assert, and most teenagers draw on such experiences to build them up, and as long as it lasts for a short time, most eventually stop painting their hair purple and piercing every area of their face when they know it annoys you; and if it's not in the appearance, then it shows up in thoughts and actions, where they defy anything and everything just to be difficult. You see, they know what a nightmare they are making your life, and the more critical and disempowering you are to them, the more the rebellion. Remember, they are trying to be an adult from a childlike state, so they actually don't know how or what to do with this bubble of power that can be upheld with gushing hormones in their bodies. The natural response is usually that most parents roll their eyes or speak to their partners about it, and they try to reason with them to get them to see logic, giving valid reasons why they should be listening to their parents—because they know what's best for them, right?

Wrong!

Leave them alone; it's falling on deaf ears. They need to know that you love them unconditionally. Focus on all the other bits about them, through which they are not voicing rebellion. Don't unconsciously reward the rebellion, especially if you don't like what you see.

For them, it is a way of understanding things and how they fit in life and the world, which is why we see it typically in toddlers, and then in teenagers, and for some, it lasts their entire life! This brings me to the point of rebellion that actually then gets in the way—your way.

Think about rebellion with the obvious culprit: food, especially healthy food, or messages on exercise or health, and every bit about it that's good. You end up doing the opposite. When everyone is eating a good wholesome meal, you desire to prove a point and order the unhealthiest pizza meal going, and then you gloat just to see their faces. There are all sorts of situations with alcohol and drugs, and disrupted sleep patterns, when rebellion is played out. The thing is that these are obvious facets of rebellious behaviour. It's the hidden patterns of communication in adults—the stimulus and the response. Rebellion is an active power, and whilst many know its impact, when it comes to unhealthy living, that force is very powerful in the moment especially when the communication takes your actions away from good healthy habits so do watch that and observe these patterns in yourself. So why do that? Because they can feel something powerful within themselves, and that it can attract attention to themselves.

They don't want to be Goody Two Shoes, so they go to the opposite side. It's a different energy, and it depends on which side was rewarded. I have more on this, further along in this book.

You cannot reason with this rebellion, and it's actually hard work being with someone that displays it for the worst whilst it is going on. This rebellious nature of your inner child can be played out at any age. Obviously, we would expect it when you are actually a child, but if rewarded wrongly, this will risk a communication pattern conditioned into their adult life.

I suppose it is an attitude, and you have to think about when this is displayed—when are you stubborn when it comes to your health? When you know you need to do or be a certain way in order to live healthily, what stops you that is rebellious in nature?

What age do you go back to then?

An adult ego state is when there are internal resources of reasoning and insight at play, and being mindful and present in that moment. In comparison, when your rebellious child ego is in play, your internal resource becomes limited in terms of your thought and range of emotions. This impacts your actions next, what you do and don't do.

From my perspective, I love rebellion, and I love to challenge the status quo, as long as it's done mindfully and in my adult ego state; so that would be the equivalent of a positive rebellion ego state. I love witnessing children saying NO at times to parents, to teachers, or to other people, where they know the truth and disagree using their intuitive reasons. It does not serve us to live in and within the confines of fear and rules. Health today is confusing and over-complicated, its messages controlled and delivered through a network that has reasons to encourage illness rather than wellbeing. I am saying no to being influenced by outdated ways to be healthy, and to a disjointed system of information! Enough! We all need to be owning and developing our own health and wellness, and this book gets you to see all the different integrated angles in order to do so.

Question for you:
"When are you triggered to be unhelpfully rebellious?"

Guiding principle:
"The unhelpful rebellion is part of your child ego state, and needs careful management, or it will get powerfully out of control."

Rebellion Within You – The Good Part

As a child in Africa, during feeding times, I remember that my parents (and in particular, my mum) and grandparents would insist that I finish my food on my plate during meal times. My mum constantly reminds me to this day what a nightmare I was during feeding times. You see, her peer and circle of influence happened to be my grandparents, and they insisted she needed to feed me more because I was too skinny, and people were talking because I was the first born; and at that time, being fed well and looking plump was a sign of health, good living, and prosperity.

The truth was that I was incredibly healthy, strong and able, and just very active. Food was the last thing on my mind; I would eat what I needed and that's all, and I never once had any fear of saying no to anyone about anything I did not want to do. Don't be a "yes" slave; learn when to say no, in a way that is positive for you. My saying "no" to too much food was a healthy rebellion against someone who thought they knew better than me, but that positive rebellion was not through a conditioned thought process taught on how to be; it came from my powerful intuitive child voice. With awareness even as a small kid, I knew my body and the feeling of fullness or the sheer lack of interest in food, which for many parents cannot be understood. Their focus is how to nurture their children. The concept of over nurturing does not come to mind. Overfeeding may not be done in one sitting, but constant offerings of food and drink can teach a child to graze and overeat that way. You see, for my younger self, my need for food was a physical need rather than an emotional one. Like me, no kid would willingly starve themselves, as long as there is no medical or clinical issue.

Children who have the confidence and perspective to say no to anything unjust or unfair in, say, a school environment, or to the teachers that are directing power control, are ones we need to watch—their perspectives are important and very valid, and they may just go on to become important people that change the course of history for the better. They may be our next generation change makers, as long as they are nurtured to use that perspective for their whole time. We just need to think about some famous and inspiring people who did not settle for the easy way—they knew and continued to believe in their ideas, and they rebelled against the norm—and changed the status quo of impossible to possible. Look at how Thomas Edison and Einstein worked.

Rebellion, when used positively, challenges and shifts perspectives. It can be a level of assertiveness and aliveness—a form of resonance, a set of inherent skills to question and be curious. So it's not that such personalities are disruptive; they need to be shown the correct manner in which to voice their opinion, rather than be told not to voice it at all, and instead to be quiet and compliant. How can that be good for their health? It just says to them that their voice doesn't matter and needs to be silenced in order to have good manners, which can have a huge impact on their confidence and self-esteem and as they grow. They only need to go on and find a repeat experience of the same or similar before it becomes a stubborn core belief about themselves, and that their voice does not matter and is better shut off and silenced. What we need to teach our young is that we are all unique and can accept and be included, and that there is value to us all. That is what we now miss in education and other similar institutions.

It is therefore important to have them "feel" that they are heard, and to acknowledge their important perspectives. They are not always after agreement. They need to learn that everyone has the right to express their perspectives in an open, honest manner, and as long as that starts very early on, then it is usually that we have a thorough grounding on our functional existence and safe survival within the family pack and wider society. It can start at any stage in life, but imagine if we could start young, and how resilient and happy and skilled they would be. I know many parents who, without the knowledge of coaching, have tackled such issues, and with very positive outcomes, which they have also transferred into their workplace with colleagues, peers, and teams, as well as with friends and relatives. So, it is an all-encompassing way of getting to a more positive and consistent result. The danger is always with the person that cannot take a no!

Have you ever been on a diet and have decided on an eating regime, and then you go out with friends; only you are okay with what you choose, but they are not, and they try to convince you to stop or change just for today—their happiness depends on what YOU eat, right?

Think about it; their happiness depends on you making yourself unhappy, breaching your own contract, or even losing a value like integrity with yourself. At this stage, either have an adult conversation with your friends or ditch them.

At times, let's take pleasure in people who have another perspective. It is about keeping an open mind and allowing learning and new knowledge to take shape from the place of understanding, growth, and awareness. It is useless just taking on information without the next steps—how it fits or sits with you, and crucially any resulting implementation.

If there is no container for such perspectives in people, then they become different, challenged, and certainly not all together. We need to allow this space for each of us at any age. Expect rebellion in teenagers; it is a hormonal, physiological pattern that directly has a hit on their behaviour. It is all about the next stage of making sense of the world and, in particular, how they fit in, in a way that is unique but also in a way that develops good relationships with people. They are growing up, and it's very important to let them do just that. Over-engineering will get you and them in trouble. Get out of the way and just watch; be there for them if they need that, but let them ask for help first.

Question for you:
"When can you use the active and powerful positive rebellion when it comes to your health?"

Guiding principle:
"Say yes to yourself, and no to anything or anyone
that takes you away from your goals to start with,
until you get so skilled that saying yes still works out for you
because you are able to manage yourself beautifully."

Attention-Seeking Antics

You would think that this behaviour belongs to children—and mostly it does—as they navigate through those early years to work out what's what, and how they fit in with the bigger picture and what their relationships mean; testing them is a necessary evil. This can also be displayed by adults because, somewhere within them, there is a part that has not been heard or validated or even discovered. But this supposed "neediness" is a way of checking in with things every now and again—to see that you exist! In part, you may only engage in activities and behaviour patterns that do get a response from people in ways that are sometimes expected and sometimes not. It is also debatable as to whether this so-called "demand" for attention is the best way to check in.

Let's not confuse the fact that demand for attention is necessary when, say, you break a leg or get hungry or feel unsafe, as there are some legitimate reasons to get the attention. This is not something that is generally problematic. What I am talking about is the emotional check-in—the "I exist" piece—it is a basic survival instinct for humans, who are like pack animals and are best nurtured in social groups. However, today, we have so much more to do and be, and really find it very difficult to spin so many plates and keep them all equally in motion without a few crashing in front of us. Yes, life today is a little more challenging in terms of navigating your way through some basics; and in a way, that is both balanced and meaningful.

The way we live out our lives has a connection to past experiences and, in particular, childhood experiences.

If that is built up to be healthy and within a wholesome framework, even with challenges, and as long as there was the right conversation, support, and openness to build up resilience, strength, and confidence for those and future challenges, then we would not use attention seeking tactics so much. There is, however, a fine line between what is right and what becomes needy and self-imploding.

I would say that for those who are "attention seeking" in an unhelpful way, usually perceive themselves and the world a little differently, even in a little uncertain way, and you would not know it if you saw them. They hold down great jobs and even have social variety in terms of friendships and other relationships; however, at times, they show this behaviour, especially when challenged in a certain way or by someone or an aspect of their life. In my experiences, this type of personality can use their lack of health as their way of attention seeking. The changes that they need to make get sabotaged by themselves. They get a lot of attention for not taking good care of themselves, and they attract "rescuers." They blame circumstances and people, and do it in quite a dramatic way. They don't get the results they want because they never get started, or if they do, they don't continue, because they don't think they can, and they think of every excuse they can find to justify it. They still blame someone else for their defeats. As health is about change and embracing the evolving philosophies of best practice and a deeper understanding of yourself, this can be enough to encompass this train of behaviour, because they usually hit a wall!

It usually needs some kind of trigger and timing for this to show itself, and it is unpredictable. You cannot guess it. It is a psychological game albeit unconscious. Any negative outcome with their health is one of many triggers.

So, what is attention seeking really, and does it serve us at all? Dysfunctional attachment in early years can lead to many unhelpful traits later on in life and my observations with some negative attention seeking traits and negative rebellion is that it can be linked.

Again, it's a way of ensuring our survival—that we exist, that we are important, that we need recognition conditionally and uncondit-ionally. Babies and smaller children are very in tune with this technique of survival; they will cry and behave in ways that will create attention for their needs to be met. When you give appropriate attention to the need (e.g., "change my nappy" or "I need feeding" cries), and once dealt with, the baby stops and is satisfied and happy again. However, when the one true need—this can be physical or emotional—is ignored or dealt with inappropriately, despite the baby getting louder and louder in their plea for attention, what then?

Well, as any parent knows in the early days of having a baby, it is about dealing with so many things, and getting to know your baby and dealing with their cries through a process of elimination. I have changed nappies when my babies were actually hungry, and vice versa!

Sometimes we reward ways for attention seeking that then become counterproductive. Remember, I raised the principle of rebellion or compliance in everyone's nature through ego states. What triggers one or the other can be different, but negative rebellion can also be linked with attention seeking and how these become manifested through time, paying attention specifically here not to babies but to the adult population.

This power balance moves from "requesting attention" to "wanting attention," and they quickly and creatively learn how to gain attention "on demand" in a dysfunctional way.

We need to be careful how this so called "game" plays out, because much human behaviour is learnt and conditioned for rewards, so if inappropriate attention is demanded and gets rewarded, then it will get repeated and demanded. When there is a lack of something emotional or physical, what happens is that the behaviours become a vehicle for the "lack."

This can become a dysfunctional relationship with self, and does not serve the greater good of the person or the people in their company.

Let me give you an example of someone who wanted to lose weight to save her marriage—at least in her perception. She saw good results, and she was happy with her weight loss and the attention she was getting again from her husband, who she claimed was being very encouraging and supportive. That kept her motivated to continue. However, after a few months, what she noticed was that her husband, who she was counting on to encourage her, was otherwise engaged in his work; and as that took over, she experienced a decrease in his attention toward her and what she was accomplishing. I ask you to not make an opinion of her, whether critical or sympathetic.

If you have ever tried losing excess weight, you know that it is not easy, and whilst motivation and hopes are high at the beginning, if you have a lot to lose, it can feel never-ending. It's great at the start because motivation and hope are high, and then once you are somewhere in the middle, it feels like an eternity and you need support—all kinds of support—and that is okay and mostly appropriate.

But back to her example:

Helen felt a little lost and somewhat betrayed and disappointed because she had aligned her weight loss goal to save her marriage. She was doing something to save it whilst her husband just carried on as normal. Her motivation dwindled.

Her words: "Well, he is not paying me any attention anymore. It's like he doesn't care about the way I look, so why should I bother? It's too hard anyway, and I can't do it anymore."

Luckily, she carried on a little more, and she became hostile—"the hell with him"—but she was going to do it regardless! Except one weekend, her need for this attention played out in an unhelpful and irrational way. Will, her husband, got himself a promotion at work, and he brought home some good wine, chocolate, and their favourite cake to help celebrate. She immediately flipped and shouted at him, saying how bad he had been in supporting her, that she was on a diet and she could not eat that, and why would he want to ruin it for her, and that he doesn't love her. The accusations just flowed out like verbal diarrhoea.

He, of course, was shocked by it all and tried to reason with her and keep his composure. I personally don't think it was sabotage on his part; he just did not think it through properly. And yes, he admitted that it was not helpful at that moment. She, of course, refused to accept his apology, was very emotional, and kept relentlessly pitching to fight with him, completely dismissing his promotion.

Can you see how desperate she is for attention, for love, to be seen, to be heard, to be valued?

Can you see how quickly she was triggered back to her childlike self, and yet her real age was 45?

Can you see that this was not just about the cake and wine, but that it was a pitch for many years of not dealing with whatever needed to be dealt with, such as unresolved conflict?

She went into victim mode, where she felt sorry for herself, and she was persecuting him for his actions relentlessly. It was like war between "I am right; you are wrong," and despite his sincere apology, this was still not enough for her.

His response was, "Okay, that's fine; you don't have to eat it—it is not a big deal." And he poured himself a glass of wine and tucked into his piece of cake and chocolates without her, and was quite happy.

She then watched him eat and drink in front of her, whilst pacing up and down the lounge, getting more and more agitated and angry at what she saw. There was bitterness. She held out for 6 hours before she decided to eat the rest of what was left, which was three quarters of the cake, chocolate, and almost half the bottle of wine, and basically swallowed it and said to him: "See what you have done now!"

This is game-playing at its best, a dramatic set of events that did not need to happen this way at all, and yet it is not the first and won't be the last, and there are people playing this out to a lesser or greater extent in so many of life's events all over the world. There is a great deal of discounting and, for many, this is the way they live out their lives, in desperation, for attention and to fill holes that are lacking in something so important to them.

This marriage could not work in its present way, but it did not need to end. This could have been saved and put on a much better footing. Her need for attention went back to her childhood, and the game playing was a strategy in her adult life. What she needed and what she did do was to account for her needs, and share her vulnerability and what she wants for her happiness for now and her future, and that will allow her to be more transparent with her thoughts and full range of emotions.

They are very much together today and have saved the way they communicate with each other, with more understanding, kindness, and love; she learned how to do that, and he was, of course, immensely grateful that he got a happier woman.

This example also makes another important point: getting healthy, and in this case, losing weight to save a marriage. When two parties are not engaged in the overall goal, it will not happen and is unsustainable, and it makes way for self-sabotage and psychological games. Changing health for yourself is first and foremost, and you will see what a difference that makes in terms of your own empowerment. So many people make goals that are not for themselves, but they associate these goals with someone or something else, without dealing with the core problem of what is really going on.

Question for you:
"What aspect of life triggers you to be needy
and seeking emotional attention?"

Guiding principle:
"Game playing is never going to end well;
instead name what is going on, get to the core of the problem,
and deal with it rationally."

Fussy

Another area I have come across many times is when parents ask me about the fussy-eating children. Being fussy can be more of a psychological need than a physical dislike to something. Eating is meant to be a positive social activity, but when the correct environment is not created to eat and be together, problems do occur. If there is too much force given to your children to eat green beans, for example, they can grow up really disliking green beans, and actually a whole array of vegetables, and they become fussy. This establishes, in many cases, an unhelpful relationship with the idea of this kind of food, and we know that vegetables of all colours, varieties, and textures are important for our nutritional needs. So, this can pose a threat of under-nourishment, and the potential for disease in some eaters.

If you think about it, there is a lot of drama around eating certain things, or not, in some cases, that gives fuel to the potential of attention-seeking behaviours, because kids tend to know very quickly what it is that they do that gets them the attention, even if the attention is bad, as in punishment or being told off for something. Sometimes some parents only communicate to their children when the children are being told to do something they don't want to, or when they are genuinely being critical to them. When a child does something like sitting quietly and reading, it's quite normal to let it be, and because parents now need the peace, they are afraid to disrupt it; so they go quiet and just let it be, sometimes missing the need for acknowledging the exact behaviour they are happy with, and the silence or lack of acknowledgment can be as non-rewarding.

So, be absolutely sure to make more of a fuss about the things they do, when they happen. Be more vocal in words, body language, and tonality than when they don't do something right. I am writing another book, called *Ice Cream or Green Beans*, which is about engaging in a healthy and rewarding way to get children well-grounded and with healthy relationships with themselves, others, and food! Much of the world's epic growth of lifestyle disease and obesity can be punctured and reversed if we start here. Actually, even if you are not yet a direct parent, you will notice some childlike behaviours and ways of thinking and engaging that you can still learn from, which play out in some way that is not always of help to you in the long run. It is a fascinating take on the way we are with the choices we make. It adds yet another valuable dimension to this book, as well as standing in its own right to prevent lifestyle diseases like diabetes and obesity in our children.

Think of someone that is fussy—when did the fussiness start, and what are the actual characteristics and trigger traits of it? How does it start and end? What happens in the middle of the episode? Is it an acute episode, or has it become chronic and something that is repeated? Look and observe, and then think about what gets thrown at it in terms of problem solving. How much attention is given to it? How does it make the individual feel during and after such episodes?

So, back to "fussy" as a challenge from within. Think about when they say they don't want to eat this or that—what happens? What alternatives are provided, if any, or do they just stay hungry because mum and dad insist on being "right" and "winning."

I know when my children were little, I had to deal with my children's battle with some foods, but for some reason, it was the opposite of what most other children did like eating like bread, pasta, and potatoes. Mine ate greens to their hearts content. I was relentlessly fighting against that and their strong minds just because I was told that its things like pasta, bread that fill their tummies, or I would make it a nightmare for myself, thinking that they would just be hungry, and I kept demanding that they eat the food, and the kitchen was the last place I wanted to tie myself down to for longer than needed. I also did not want to give them rice every day; I wanted their palette to accept and enjoy a variety of tastes and textures. I fought on and completely dismissed the good that was going on: They ate up all their vegetables and fruits, and they loved salads—raw at that!

It was only one day, when I finally woke up and got out of my own head, that I actually saw with immense clarity how lucky I was that every child in my house had been eating foods that were healthy and wholesome. I also understood that quite rightly they just did not like some foods or were not hungry. I missed all these cues from them, and that is understandable when I just wanted to protect and do the best for them. We have a huge part to play in developing our self-awareness, and even parents who think they know everything there is to know, don't—they can't ! We evolve through learning and from experience.

Even with mealtimes, I remember thinking, "Well, I have cooked it now, so it must be eaten." To request self-recognition with food is cultural of course, but in my culture, feeding and being fed is quite important as a way of showing love and nurturing; and mums need to feel success and achievement in this manner. They can get quite offended if you refuse their food; not because you don't like it but because of the meaning they associate with presenting a meal for their family, and most mums will be insistent and almost force you to eat it. When you say you are full, they will insist on you having more and more. Luckily, I did not get that far, but I would worry all the time that my kids were not eating properly, especially when a routine baby and child clinic was coming up monitoring their growth and weight. Mine were all really small, and other babies were putting on so much weight that they would get all the praise. I would sit there quietly, wondering what I had done wrong. My babies were small and ate small amounts of food. Please be assured that they were not forced to eat or finish things; it was me that felt sad that I could not get them to eat what and how much I wanted them to.

You would be surprised at the stories I have heard since then, about some parents' aggression and control over their children's eating habits, punishing and inducing guilt on them. For me and my experience, mealtimes just took a little longer than they needed to. It became a temporary chore rather than a pleasure, as I was conditioned for it to be. Thankfully, I learnt that whatever they did was okay, and I must have masked my inner distress well. Luckily, my children are not fussy eaters, and they do eat bread, pasta, and potatoes, but it is secondary to their love of fresh fruit and vegetables. I am so lucky; I know many parents that struggle to get any plant based foods or very little into their children's everyday eating that they have to resort to hiding it in foods, mashed in hiding the taste and texture into something that do eat or recognise or have to bribe them with ice cream. How will that ever improve plant based food education for them. It has to be an authentic sensory experience or they just won't eat when they are older. I understand how tricky it is for so many time poor parents.

Instead, let's celebrate the needs of individuals. Even as babies, they will grow and evolve, and we should instead offer fuss and recognition over the things they do by themselves, to reassure them that these are the behaviours that are acceptable and best serve them. Don't be afraid of getting it wrong, as long as you know something to correct it as soon as you become aware. It is about using your awareness and observations, and not ignoring them. That's the thing about parenting; it is all about learning, and I can now share my experiences and learning, which I hope will be of value to you or to future mums, dads, and children.

Please visit www.SanjayaPandit.com and you can register your interest at no obligation to buy my next book *Ice Cream or Green Beans*.

Question for you:
"What are you fussy about—nothing? Think again."

Guiding principle:
"There is both a healthy and unhealthy side of being fussy; the distinction between the two is your job for awareness."

You Are Your Own Worst Enemy – Self-Sabotage

Have you ever started something in your own health journey, only to give up at the first hurdle, or have you just never finished what you started in anything that is important to you or meaningful? That is a challenge that only you know about, and as much as it is easy to blame outside factors for this fact, it is actually from within. I call it self-sabotage.

Self-sabotage comes from unconscious beliefs that you may hold about yourself, others, and the world. What sabotages your health journey from within you?

Self-sabotage exists when you don't actually believe that you will get there, but on the surface, you have everything thrown at achieving it; so, sometimes the behaviours that become apparent in your goals and actions for health, are counterproductive and take you away from what you want to achieve. That's not lack of willpower as you have been told. It is sabotage and comes from a deeper setting. To understand it and tackle it, you have to go deeper to understand yourself.

Now, I know other people can sabotage things as well. Some of our relationships are built around safety and familiarity, so when someone else says something to you that discourages you in what you decide to do for yourself, remember that it's their sabotage playing out too. When we try to voice our opinions and our wisdom, there is always someone who wants to knock it down, and we start to think that we can't do it anymore—no one likes to be knocked down before they even start. I have experienced it so many times, and had to work on my own saboteurs to help me barricade myself from the outsiders.

This concept of working on yourself, to strengthen yourself, is very important, because when you do something different, or have a purpose that goes against the grain, or even if you want a better life for yourself, want to make lots of money, and move somewhere different, away from family, you can get knocked down by other people who have tried and just could not do it, so why would they ever encourage you to? If they can keep you small, they can live with themselves. So we all know there are some people who would never want you to step up. They play on your beliefs as well, and in time you can actually become them, unless you work deeper and understand the core of your sabotage. Let me tell you that the most powerful saboteurs and sabotaging behaviours and actions are beliefs taken from your loved ones—parents, sisters, brothers, close friends, and of course, yourself—and your incomplete, unsatisfied experiences. Call them naysayers if you want to; it's the same thing.

When we start to step up and claim life to its fullest, we get sabotaged, because there is a part of you that wants to be protected—close to only what you know and is familiar. Growth and learning do mean stepping into the unknown, and because that is where our true potential lies, it can be uncomfortable and therefore opens you to your own sabotage, or sabotage from others who frankly fear the change in you for themselves.

We start to listen to the voices in our heads that tell us that "we can't do it; it's too big; who do we think we are; no one likes us anyway; just get a simple job to make money." The bigger the goal and the bigger the dream, the louder, bolder, and more forceful the voices of doom. It is like a sleeping giant troll, waiting to get back to its job because, for so long, you have not done anything bold and courageous enough to wake it; but now life is such that you have heard your calling, you have been asked to step up, and you have been told to reverse some disease in you, and this troll wakes up.

Think about it; what have you tried to correct or achieve for your greater good, but still haven't? It's been labelled "for another time." (What happened? What and who got in the way?)

Another feature of self-sabotage is procrastination. Do you procrastinate? Do you put things off till tomorrow?

What is it about your health that you are putting off? How come? What's the real reason?

We are designed to be great, not just to fit in and be the same as everyone else. Some will approach their death with so much work that is incomplete, and so many life experiences that are incomplete or not even initiated.

Learn to tune out your self-sabotaging thoughts, feelings, and behaviours, and learn instead to listen to the beauty of that little voice, hidden perhaps in the background, and start giving it air time. That's the voice that knows what you are capable of for your health, because this is your window to a greater life in other areas, like work and business, entrepreneurship and leadership, family and relationships, and finance and abundance of wealth and opportunity.

I specialise in helping people with self-sabotage, whether in health, personal, or business settings. Please visit www.SanjayaPandit.com to download a free resource I use to reflect on your saboteur profiles that you can fill in for yourself. Oh Yes there can be more than one kind, some people have a committee of them getting in their way of progress. Let's get you understanding yourself a bit more, as it is only through awareness that you can change anything that may be stopping you moving forward.

Question for you:
"What do you self-sabotage repeatedly, and how?"

Guiding principle:
"This world teaches us to stay small, and that you don't deserve an abundance of whatever you desire. In the world of faith, dreams, and belief, and in the Universe—if you desire it— it's possible."

Lack of Awareness

Many of us don't know that we don't know. It is one stage of learning: unconscious incompetence. When you first started walking or riding a bike, you would have approached it as if you could do it, and it looked easy until you tried and realised that you did not know that you did not know—you were completely blind to the experience, and you stepped into the next stage of learning conscious incompetence. Now, you know that you have to learn something here, and you don't know it—it is a skill that you don't have. Many of us go through life with so many experiences, and yet it is very rare that we reflect on them to see if there is a pattern, something that the higher powers are trying to teach us in some way.

Think about it; how many women in abusive relationships find a way out with one abusive partner, and then go straight into another abusive relationship. This is the sad truth, and no one helps them really develop their learning. Finding shelters and safe houses, and providing social care, all helps of course, but who actually in that team helps these women understand what makes them tick, and what attracts those types of men to them, even though it is so sad that anyone has to go through such pain and fear. I am not saying that it is the women's fault at all, but it is a pattern for which they need help to break, and they need to start believing that they deserve better, that they can be loved and cherished, and that the trajectory they once had will start to change its course to better men. They have not learnt something important about themselves, so they do it again and again until they reach a breaking point, which forces them to reflect.

Anything that we do repeatedly and are drawn into is a pattern—a conditioning based on outdated beliefs and thoughts about ourselves and others. That is the focus, and the results come in. Many in that space that I have spoken with have admitted that they did not think they deserved anything else. Don't get me wrong; I am not saying that this is only the victim's fault, and in no way do I lessen the seriousness of abuse to victims of domestic abuse. Help them by changing their beliefs about themselves, improving their self-esteem, and making them realise that they deserve genuine love on equal terms. They need help, and so do the oppressors. There is a pattern in what we do—even unconsciously; our blind spot—and we need to look at it to see what is really in our belief system. It is only with the realisation of their self-worth that they will start to attract partners that understand their worth too, and treat them accordingly.

With most of us, in such times when we have a poor relationship with life, adding time to reflect just doesn't happen, because it doesn't always give us instant results, and we don't always like what we learn; but don't let that stop you, because it is temporary and something you have to go through to get to the other side. Having a qualified and I mean qualified professional coach or other therapist that sees your deserving potential can help you through it.

We are not taught to reflect. We just go after one thing and another, and that's it, and as long as the results come in, then great; we have nothing to reflect on, right?! It's only when things go "pop" that we start to think that we don't always have all the answers. Life is different to every single one of us. Some experience negative things when they are very young, and some experience that much later in life. We are not good at reflecting or even asking for help. We just muddle through life or go to the massive collection and range of self-development books to work through answers. It helps to a point, but self-awareness, to the degree that I am referring to, comes from deep within. That's where it is like gold, and it is precious. To reflect and get awareness of ourselves, we have to be still and quiet. How many of us can do that in a normal life on a daily basis? We don't make time or space for it, and we don't understand it's benefits. We are taught that life has to be life with a heightened adrenalin —the fight or flight response. This is what we are used to, from the moment we wake up to the moment we go to sleep, and then we do it all over again, leaving any semblance of reflection or self-awareness only for holidays—and then self-awareness only goes as far as where we should go for our next holiday! For most, we are not enlightened with real knowledge of ourselves. People actually resist sitting still and relaxing in ways that are appropriate because they just can't do it. They are even scared of self-reflection and awareness, and would resist and continue in denial, only addressing symptomatic relief on life and health.

This is why people end up leading lives that are superficial and not congruent. Things are disjointed and not connected in a way that connects you to your deeper self, of who you are and what you are born to do and be. So don't wait for the perfect anything; do it today, and start becoming aware of yourself today. Get the self-realisation earlier—imagine life with that as your true partner.

You will typically get through the first phase, which is really things you know very well and are well practiced at. It is the same thing I ask my clients to do when I ask them to set goals and aspirations, because they name the obvious ones first—you know, the information that is practiced for sharing because it is safe information, and it's still guarding you. You need to get beyond this, deeper into the layers, where you feel curious and don't recognise yourself in some way. It's really like diving into a dark cave; and yes, it is scary when done on your own. The cave lights up once you start on the self-awareness journey, but until then you will lead life like a robot—the way the world has taught you, and the way that it is accepted. Some of my clients have used a metaphor to describe awareness through coaching at a deeper level as if it was like "peeling away the layers of an onion, one layer at a time to get to your real self, at your core, hidden by unnecessary layers taken on by your life, and protected to the point that it was crippling, with an army of saboteurs controlling you at every level."

Powerful, don't you think? This is where transformation happens and you can liberate and fly high, changing the shape, dialogues, and outdated guarding systems that no longer serve you to live your best life. It's a truly remarkable experience. Everyone is deserving of this.

Get the self-awareness; do it and keep doing it! Now! put this book down and remember to come back to it; go somewhere peaceful, and reflect on your life so far. What do you want for yourself that you are denying? Close your eyes if you have to, or focus on something outside your window that is beautiful and gives you a lovely feeling.

What is your love and passion in life, and are you living it?

For bonuses go to ...

Question for you:
"What are you learning so far?"

Guiding principle:
"Self-awareness is your true life blood;
from here, learn to steer your life."

Chapter principle:
"As well as external challenges to your health, you also have your internal challenges. These are your conditioned beliefs and people that have influenced your thoughts.
For health to evolve, you have to get it to top priority and to its best form, and then you have to pay careful attention to what you think, what you say, and your behaviour."

Basic Psychological Needs
Are Not Being Met

Chapter 4
What's the REAL Problem?

Creating Fuss for a Cause

There can be two dimensions to being fussy or creating fuss. The first one is about certain standards and expectations, like choosing a restaurant that serves certain food options, or having your home look and feel a certain way. This is not the one I want to explore, because standards and reasonable expectations are normal and personal to us all, and when they are met, it ends there. This will be covered later in the book, when it comes to raising expectations and standards of health together.

For now, the "fuss" element I want to draw your attention to is the one that is played out a bit like a game of "I win, you lose," which is also used to persecute or make the other person feel guilty or insignificant, or even small. I wonder if you have ever been in the company of this type of fussy person, where nothing is good enough, everything is an ordeal, and you get the feeling that they like getting off on it too! This type of fussiness is like the attention seeking we alluded to earlier on, and I wanted to explore how it gets encouraged, created, and evolves in some people or may show up from time to time in people who are triggered or stressed out. This is an aspect of relational health that is unhealthy, and so it is an important component of the overall corrective measure we need to take for our total health. I have already mentioned that we have social behaviours and taught ideals. Good relationships add to the overall picture of our health.

I also want to reassure you that there is a much more productive, kinder, loving way to deal with what is at the heart of this type of fussiness, and how to prevent it from developing. Here are some questions to get you thinking about yourself and the people you know.

When and how do you experience fussiness, and witness it with yourself and others? Have you ever been fussy just to dig your heels in? What was the outcome? What was the real issue here?

Firstly, let's deal with how it gets rewarded, so that the actual nature and what is behind it can be uncovered. We need to remove the mask that hides the real deal behind such unhealthy behaviour.

What we witness as it develops is a strong will and desire to be right, and to cause as much commotion as is possible for yourself and others with this drama. You know, the typical experiences, like when sitting around a dinner table in disharmony because someone is labelled a fussy eater, or the time when a colleague digs their heels in just because they don't agree with something, and that gets in the way of the progress, resulting in a bad all-round feeling.

I know the ordeal many parents go through getting their kids to eat the right foods, like greens, but all they seem to want to do is eat the chips and then wonder when the dessert is coming out. But instead of ignoring this behaviour of not wanting to eat their green vegetables, what actually happens is that you create a lot of attention on the fact that they are not eating what you know is good for them, and it is that exact point in time that this fussy little eater has got you over a barrel.

The power shifts from you as a parental authority figure, to them as a kid with perceived power over you. Time evolves in this struggle, and each time, they are watching and learning everything that is being created around this fuss: replacement food being offered; punish-ment for not having their green food; talking about them to other people about their fussy profile, when they are clearly there;

deliberately paying a lot of attention to the good kids round the table who do eat their green vegetables; and ultimately labelling and calling them "fussy." It can go on and on, and even if there is no language through spoken words and your tone, there are clues in your behaviour and body language that can contribute more to that fusspot knowing that they are getting a lot of attention through this. It can certainly start giving them an identity or even a role to play out in life.

It is easily done, especially when you disconnect from that child and go into your head because you think you know best, right? You are back on your agenda because, as a parent, you have to get them to eat their vegetables, right?

Our minds can learn anything, even stuff that is not good for us to learn! Let me give you an example using my dog, because dogs can be conditioned to learn anything we teach them, through rewards, just like human brains. They will do anything to please their human owners. I remember a trainer telling me that I had, without realising, rewarded the behaviours that I did not want in my dog, who at that time was eating socks—yes, socks—falling out of our washing by mistake, or socks left outside in parks while we were training in obedience.

When Casper, our dog, was a pup, we saw him with one of our socks that had fallen out of the washing machine, and he was, and is, very very quick at retrieving items—he is, after all, a fox red Labrador retriever. With socks, however, that has become "high value" because of the panic and fuss we created in trying to get him to drop it! He now will retrieve/steal any sock, anywhere, despite the "leave it" command, which works brilliantly on everything but socks. He would put this sock in his mouth and look at us, and I would give a loud yell and then panic would set in because of my conditioning and alertness from other dog owners who had said to me, "You have a Lab; oh, they eat everything and anything, including socks... socks you have to be careful with because they can eat them and cause damage, and they can't pass through...you may get a blockage, which will mean an operation and a hefty vet bill." Well, thanks for that, I thought at the time. So when I saw that sock in Casper's mouth, I was already seeing a problem and consequences, and I saw a very large vet bill, which of course I wanted to avoid. So I panicked and called the whole troop down, and we chased him round the lounge, and he ran, and we chased him, and he would not give it up—and for some reason, he decided to swallow it! Even he did not see that coming! He won the play game.

Subsequently, many times, after he had the other socks, gloves, or whatever he found while out on walks, we just went into autopilot reaction mode and we did the same thing: chasing him, with lots of commands to drop it and leave it. He would sense the panic and concern for him, and each and every time, we rewarded this behaviour in him, when actually we were trying to stop him from harm! He learned a rewarding behaviour, and he gets lots of attention and love anyway with the correct attention when he is behaving, except for this. Now, today, he eats socks without the need for attention. Please don't worry; he is fine, and we are managing this behaviour with a good degree of success in undoing his learning, and replacing it with something a lot better, and healthier for us both! But we have to be careful with him and socks, because he still remembers and will try and push for it.

The "high value" thing with anyone that is fussy is the level of attention they get as a result of their fussiness. It establishes their existence and importance, and gives them the significance they are craving, which in their mind is lacking somewhat. Now, I will always be much better at training humans than dogs in this manner, but for those wanting to know how things worked out with Casper—who is now 5 years and just as energetic—he will still do it every now and again, but because we don't panic and create attention, and we just go about our business, he will run across us, slapping the sock firmly in his mouth from left to right, and then look at us as if he is saying, "Hey, look, I have a sock... are you going to chase me—do I have your attention?"

But we ignore it and go about our business, even with our hearts in our mouths! He loses interest because it is not getting him anything, and then he drops it and walks away most times, and we reward that instead, and we have learnt to be super quick ourselves. It is still a work in progress because he is so playful, and it is nowhere near where I would like it to be. I am definitely better at training humans than animals though, and he has shown me holes in my leadership style with him. Don't let them get the better of you, but do it in a way that is loving and not punishing, and that goes for humans too.

Labelling yourself as fussy, or others as fussy, is not the best thing to do either, because then you have to be just that, right? It becomes your identity tag, with delight at the attention it gets you! It is the people around you that are more challenged at managing such behaviour. What you created then keeps challenges you.

So, think about what fussy people are really after, and see if you can assess when this all started for them. Teaching them a more positive way to get attention for the right reasons will break down their barriers and make them believe that they don't need to create fuss to get the attention they are craving or need. Attention and recognition are the higher value treat—it is never about fruit, vegetables, fish, and meat. This type of conditioned behaviour for rewards does not just have to be around food; it can be about anything in life—types of relationships, certain work conditions—but it is high maintenance and very tiring.

Points on rewards, attention, and recognition are made throughout the book, and the difference between the healthy and unhealthy sides of them are pointed out. Keep this in your mind and memory whilst you read on.

The following is an example of a severe case, and how I found that the mind can manifest a physical reaction. What we do is to react to the symptom.

I worked with a woman, Pauline, who came to me for health coaching, and she said that she was a fussy eater. However, whilst initially talking to her about how I could help her, and about my eating programme, she did not feel confident that my programme would work well for her. She said that the sight, smell, and touch of fruit and vegetables would make her gag and feel sick, and she would have to walk away. She couldn't touch, smell, or look at vegetables, and did not eat them at all. She spent most of her salary on packaged food that was heavy in refined carbohydrates, and processed meats with artificial ingredients, which also contributed massively to her health problems, not just physically but also mentally, but she had not joined those dots as being the root cause of her problems.

So when she came to me, she was severely undernourished in key nutrients, and she felt that her body had shut down. She specifically chose me because I deal with health wholly in a connected way, and my model of coaching the Co-Active way is profound in getting results. She was so keen on it, and she got more than she bargained for. She thought about going to a nutritionist, but she felt this would be limited and have a forced approach to tackle foods she did not like, without having the headspace to have a go. She said that the sight, smell, and touch of vegetables and fruit would make her gag and feel sick, and she would have to walk away. She could not touch, smell, or look at vegetables, and had to ask someone else to shop for her for other foods if she could not go online. But still, her foods were only packaged foods, which were heavy in refined carbohydrates, processed meats, and artificial ingredients; and this also meant that she became fat and very undernourished. She wanted to move forward, mentally, physically, and spiritually. Having her as a client was hard, and I knew I had to start with her deeper fears and beliefs, but she challenged me every time, throwing curve balls about food.

Although she found me and not the other way round, she would dismiss anything I would say about good food, like throwing me a challenge so that I could also do what she has always done with people—challenge them. So I asked her what the real reason was that she had come to me.

There was a lot of resistance and tightly sewn up layers of protection.

This is an extract from the initial chemistry session we had together.

Her answer and resulting dialogue:

Pauline: "You are strong, and I have heard so much good about you, but I don't think you can help me—not really!"

Me: "So, why are you here then, as it seems you have made your mind up—have you?"

Pauline: "I don't know."

After some more questions and sometimes silence between us, and acknowledgement:

Me: "I am going to stick around whether you need my help or not."

She smiled, teared up, and her shoulders and facial tension dropped to a more relaxed state, as she realised that I meant it, and that I had gotten to one of her problems.

Unlike her previous attempts at finding a suitable coach, therapist, and all sorts of practitioners, she would challenge them so much that they could not maintain the relationship, and she reinforced that she was too fussy for people to stick around for! So, where the fussiness got her the attention, this now turned people off, and she kept testing their strength.

So I had to be quite hard, listen to my intuition, and cut through her layers whilst reassuring her that I was with her every step of the way. When she teared up, I asked her about her tears and if she thought she was ready to do the work with me. Thank goodness, she said yes, and we designed a working alliance.

But my hunch was that it was not the only thing going on, and that she had layers of troubles and protective measures taken on through life, which she needed to shed, perhaps one piece at a time; and so we agreed to investigate and learn about what was going on for her with this vegetables and sickness deal she had going on. I asked her what happened when she was younger, perhaps even in childhood. I asked what her experience was with fruit and vegetables at home or school, and at friend's houses and out with family.

The good news was that she did not need any mental health intervention or counselling as suggested by so many. She was not bulimic or had an eating disorder or needed hypnosis. She had tried them all, so why could she not get to this point with them that she wanted?

What she wanted was to move forward in a non-judgemental and authentic way. What she did ask for was to go forward, and through trusted coaching and space, with some work needed for healing of trauma as a child in this area, she was able to deal with those experiences and move forward with her eating.

So we began the work. What I learnt was that her reaction to fruit and vegetables, in a physical way of being sick and actually vomiting, was through a battleground at the dinner table when her parents insisted that she eat all her greens and the limited fruit that they did get in the household. She was pushed to sit and eat it despite her better judgement, and she would be gagging and trying not to throw up because she did not like the taste and texture of this group of foods. Her experience was not positive, and it was a punishing ritual for everyone. Her brother and sisters, of course, ate everything—they dared not leave anything! Her parents insisted that she would have to eat them, as they were good for her. They meant well, like so many do, but were completely ignorant of the harm this sort of pressure can cause. They were like many parents: so attached to their agenda that they could not see it from the other person's struggle. I did not judge her parents, and I asked her to forgive them as she is no longer that child and has real choices as an adult.

Imagine living like that! With Pauline, and many like her, that kind of childhood experience can get internalised, and those experiences say something about you. That is in fact not true, but in Pauline's eyes, it was. She made meaning of it about herself and others, especially authority figures.

She now eats greens to her heart's content, and has lost enough weight for her to feel happy and healthy, but maintains her idea that she likes to be different but is no longer desperate! She loves orange hair!

As a parent myself, I have resorted to various tactics of bribery and emotional blackmail to get my children to eat what and how much I wanted them to, but I never really struggled to get my kids to eat healthy and wholesome food. For me, it was more the portions and "finishing everything up on your plate" messages, until I learnt to stop that kind of command. All anyone wants is to get pleasure and goodness from food.

However, I know that when your child is not eating anything green at all, it becomes a concern and a mother's anguish, and then it becomes a battleground to get them to eat what we know is good for them. Children who are in families with siblings are still individual, and you will see different personalities, likes, and dislikes. So any pressure in getting children to do things they don't want to do, in a forceful way— and remember, the children can perceive force, even in a subtle way, if you think it is—is of concern and very counterproductive long term. Again, in my book, *Ice Cream or Green Beans*, we discuss these issues with clear strategies that can be applied right from the beginning.

Any dysfunctional and repetitive behaviour has a reason to exist. To move forward, you will need to deal with the real cause, however uncomfortable.

Question for you:
"Have you ever judged fussy people?"

Guiding principle:
"Fussiness is not always about self-gratification; it can in some instances be a cry for help or even a way to assert oneself—be kind and understanding, and find out what makes this trait in them."

Desperate to Be Unique and Different

Does society really celebrate difference? Think about our schooling system and how when you show a different way of thinking or doing or solving a problem; the teachers are quick enough to bring you in line with the mass indoctrination, even when your contribution and way is brilliant. I see the need to be different as having a creative force behind it. I see a diamond in a child who knows how to say, "No, my way is this." The need to be different shows up in all sorts of ways: shyness, exuberance, standing their ground, voicing expressions assertively and with confidence, and through clothes and hair.

Thinking differently can be the genius in you, especially if that thinking comes from a higher brain. Many of our inventions that we enjoy and sometimes take for granted, were born and actioned from such minds.

One of the aims of this book is to give permission to our differences, and indeed, therefore, our uniqueness, so that we can open up new perspectives from limited ideas of sameness in mass. Health is individual and creates a potential in each of us that is also unique and individual. Most will turn a blind eye to the opportunity they have every day, and join the parties that just go round and round doing the same thing and expecting different results. Is that not a definition of madness or insanity?

This is an example of what happens to us when our own identity and functioning becomes so indoctrinated and unhealthily fearful of change, that we have no space left for acceptance and compassion for any differences in people. It is never about right or wrong, and more about just being, except we make anything that impacts us right or wrong when we have narrow perspectives.

This is an example that still infuriates me, but I had to share it as it makes my point here so apt!

A group of eight friends met every month for dinner and beers. This was their normal practice throughout their adult lives, and the average age of the men was 40 years. However, one of them had decided to go vegan for health reasons, which meant that his normal steak and chips was out of the question from now on. He did wonder whether he should warn them, but decided that they would be supportive and that it would not matter. They were, after all, really good friends. What he did do for this self-care effort was to eat something before meeting them, as he knew that the venue would not be too vegan-friendly, and he may end up having plate of chips and salad.

When he told them that he had gone vegan, and that the menu was restricted so he wouldn't order—but that he was happy to get some drinks, and they could go ahead and order as normal—he was shocked at their response and opinions. In his own words, he said, "It was like grown men going backwards in age and having their dummy taken off them." They moaned, accused him of being taken in with the vegan fad thing, and they became very hostile, implying that the group ritual was interrupted and disrupted, making him feel guilty. And throughout the evening, they would offer him steak, checking if he would cave in to the pressure. He did not, of course, and kept really calm. He did feel unsupported and discouraged from his chosen path to better health for himself, and he rightly challenged them and asked the question of what the purpose of the get together was then for. Was it only about the steak and beer, or was it instead about catching up and sharing companionship with each other as they evolve through life? They had after all connected to each other through relationship problems and money deficits, and celebrated business success, travel, and so on, through time.

The following month, he decided to seek a restaurant that satisfied everyone, including him. They agreed and met again. Everyone ordered: seven steaks and one vegan meal. The others all complained about how bad the steak was and that the other restaurant was better. Again, one person who seeks to be a little different in his outlook on life was the "disruptor." in this case going vegan. It got to the stage that the other seven decided to change the meeting to another time that did not include their vegan buddy. Can you imagine how that felt? His turning vegan was so important for him that he felt it best to withdraw from the group without a fight. He did and found his own troop. The others have gone back to what they know, and are very comfortable, even though they are not in the best health themselves.

That's the problem; we are prepared and open to discussing money problems, relationship problems, and even careers, but health is difficult, which is why those that embark on getting healthier are just judged and can therefore feel alone. We all need inclusivity whilst keeping our uniqueness and different desires. Why is that so hard?

You may have experienced something similar or been in a group that could not accept something different about you. If you are going against the grain in some way, it's new, and some people will want to do is knock it down, sabotage it, or voice their opinions in such a way that it affects your belief in it. By all means, let them express their views; you owe them that, but by all means, listen to their perspective but keep yours. Have the correct boundaries in order to keep your resolve and be included in their groups, and if they still can't be inclusive and supportive, then give them a break for a while; instead, find new and more supportive people to connect with. It's not selfish—it's smart because you are trying to be the best version of yourself.

Question for you:
"What have you tried to change in your health that was difficult?"

Guiding principle:
"Have a go, again and again if you have to; your way is unique to you, and so that is important to acknowledge."

Distraction Tactics Stop You From Getting Help

This is a clever and creative tactic to take the attention away from what's really going on. It is a coping strategy to start with, which when overused, in time, becomes conditioned into a behaviour pattern that may be more troublesome than the issue that was being avoided in the first place.

At times, the person using seemingly distractive tactics may not be fully aware of what is going on for them, but if you get a hunch, and your intuition speaks to you about something, then it is usually correct and worth being a little more curious about to find out what it's trying to tell you, regarding the other person.

Many experiences with people over the years, with different ailments, led me down a more curious path. An example of what I mean by "distraction" is a classic example of a commonality in unhealthy and seriously overweight people—who I have had the honour and pleasure to work with.

My reflections on them was that the general pattern seemed to reveal a conflict in them from within, and I saw firsthand how they made themselves ironically so visible when all they wanted to do was actually hide. The worst of it was that they did not think well of themselves because of things that happened through past events—trauma in some cases, and events going back to childhood— which all resulted in feeling worthless and developing a low self-esteem. They would be just as happy to dig a hole and bury themselves in it, with a sign: "Do not find me; I am okay hiding—really, I am!"

The inner conflict arises because there is no human destined to play small, especially when their unfounded mission or purpose is trying to find its way out. We are, after all, all connected with love for ourselves and others. Your spirit tries to emerge to connect you to your higher purpose. In many cases, this conflict between your mind, body, and spirit gets you confused. We do not understand the psychology of health or ill health, and loved ones are ill equipped to deal with things with care and support, trying to find only physical symptoms that may not exist as yet. It can be a real mix of emotions, and the behaviour patterns are bizarre, with some very testing times; and because we don't always understand things, we just learn to package it all up, put it away, and do whatever we need to do in order to stay in that place, or we perceive to move forward but in an unsustainable way. It can be uncomfortable and yet so comforting to just stay in one place. Many overeaters eat more, not because they are hungry but because they are trying to deal with things not fully understood within themselves, and the eating becomes a compulsion and coping mechanism. Therefore, throwing physical exercise and nutrition at them is pointless and hard work. There is nothing about it that they don't know. Educating the educated, like in so many of today's health policies and directives, is a fundamental flaw and a waste of time and money.

Over time, and with repetitive dysfunctional strategies, this evolves into a deep and secretive hiding place from the world. Their desire to go on and off diets was a balancing mechanism—yes, I will give them that—and you know me, I like balance. The weight loss part was the positive force that had courage and safety at its heart, a point to start again, to forgive and move forward. The holding or regaining of weight was the part of fear of change, fear of the unknown, the visibility and thus attention, and denial and living with the paranoia of people who may be able to figure them out—the real them (this being the unreal perception of themselves), and their desire to protect and hide a feeling of some trauma or emotion that has still not been processed. They cannot, therefore, ever move forward, unless they are first supported in a collaborative way.

You can now imagine the difficulty as to why it is so hard to lose weight for some people, which most fitness professionals and nutritionists have no idea about. How can they connect with people, with good intentions, when they have never been in that place, or even been fat for that matter?

It's very important not to judge and make assumptions on health, and therefore ill health with people who are fat or thin, because you cannot ever know. But health and ill health is the thing **I know** so well, and it astounds me how people can find ways of hiding the truth, be in denial, and use strategies to avoid accountability and responsibility. I know, for a time, I did just that, even though it was not in my conscious awareness.

Health is complex, but it can be simplified, and when we try to fix one thing without paying attention to the other key areas, it is not sustainable, and it's the sustainability that gives us the chance to uplevel to better and better health, until you reach optimal health. The health industry is made up of so many gurus, each doing their little bit. Part of the problem from a customer's point of view is that when you fix one thing, you have another problem that now needs addressing. The private healthcare system actually mirrors the public healthcare system, in that each thing is labelled; and instead of collaborating, they tend to protect our little piece. Your health cannot transform with missing links, and because each individual healthcare business has been told only to focus on their one thing, it has become disjointed. Most have no credibility on what they say. You would expect young people, who are on Instagram promoting their exercise routines for weight loss or fitness, to be fit (of course, they are; they are young) and not have too many demands on their lives. In saying that, I also do celebrate that so many young people can inspire their own age group to stay healthy. The match between the person behind the business and the majority audience has to be correct.

Before I decided to lose weight myself, for myself, I had asked for a local personal trainer to help me get to a better size. I enjoyed all my sessions, and he really put me through my paces. I became fitter and was strict with my eating regime that he had made for me. Despite sticking to it to the letter, and after a good few years and quite a substantial payout to him, my weight did not drop. I was not getting what I asked for, and every time we had this conversation about why, he questioned me in terms of my eating and that I was putting in too many calories. It was only a few years later that I realised that his advice did not work for me and my body, and there were many at my age that were experiencing the same with him. He was a good guy, but he had devised a programme based on theory and some practice, mainly on himself. In effect, I and so many others with him at the time were his guinea pigs. You see, there was a pattern; he was getting results with young people in their 20s, but I was over 40 then, had four small children, and a business and a home to run. My daily patterns were completely different to his. He was very young, had a girlfriend, and would go to work in a public gym—and really, that's about it. His focus was purely on his personal training business, training himself and keeping fit, and reading and researching, but if he could have devised a programme from the experience of a dad, or someone lacking sleep, or someone who could eat what they wanted to, or have time at convenience, he may have realised that this programme he had devised would not work for that reality. Personal training and nutritional programmes are too simplistic and only run on the calories in and calories out principle, with fat-burning muscle work. As much as his intentions were good and hopeful, to correct health or weight takes a little more than just theory. If you want someone from the outside to help you, ask them of their experience in what they can prove, how their experience of ill health was transformed back to health, and what skills they have, and challenge the mismatch between them and their audience needs—the social and cultural demographics. In my professional view, there is a handful of people from across the world that I would pay huge respect to in the field of health and wellbeing. The rest, frankly, have just found a way to make some money, and they lack the wisdom, breadth, and depth of experience and knowledge in the way that will help you— the balanced, whole you.

This is fundamentally why I chose to qualify for my coaching credentials; I coach the whole of you, and all my programmes seek to do this, whether you are changing through an individual session or through groups. I look for balance and imbalance, and in this way we can create change. I am saying that all the answers are within you, and all my integrative coaching programmes seek for you to be in charge of yourself, who you want to be, and how you want to be. It may be that you are hiding, and the tactics you use just shut down your own inner intelligence. Stop that. I have witnessed that in myself, some years back, and used all sorts of distractive mechanisms to avoid stepping out and up with courage. Now, I am not the finished article, and neither do I want to be; life and health for me is still evolving, and will continue to do so, but it gives me something truly unique—a connection to your evolvement—and this makes us relatable to each other. It's more than enough—I am on fire, on purpose, and in charge of myself.

I am very confident in saying that many, if not all, lifestyle diseases are due to an imbalance of good consistent daily living, and an imbalance of one of the three dimensions that make us whole: mind, body, and spirit. Exploration and curiosity in ourselves are a great starting point, and we can truly understand cause and effect by digging a little deeper, peeling off the layers, and not being afraid of showing our true desires and strengths, or our passions or even our vulnerability. The only thing you need is a mirror—a coach, or a coach-type of person—to help you process the information, hold the space for you, and help you articulate information that becomes visible and felt. We are human beings who become blind and deaf, and distraction is one way you were taught to sideline yourself.

Change can only come from the foundation and acceptance of truth— real truth.

Question for you:
"What distracts you from getting yourself on a better footing?"

Guiding principle:
"Let me cut to the chase: drop the excuses,
and pay full attention in understanding the real you."

Lack of Inclusion and Belonging

I got you to think about the desire to be different so that you can attain your own unique and individual character. However, in today's world, it is better and easier to join in than stand out. Standing out can be lonely, and it's difficult not to feel isolated. People who are not self-aware and have not committed to leading their mission in life, would find this hard. Self-development and learning about yourself is not grasped even when you go through experiences that are there to teach you about yourself. You knock them down, step over them, and treat them as bad luck experiences, and with a swift pat on the back—"there, there"—you go about your business, completely ignorant of the opportunity that just passed by. We are conditioned in society to be likeable and to be liked, even if it compromises what we stand for in life. That cannot be healthy long term, so watch out for what your relationships are made up of. If you want to feel included, but it's at a compromise or you are afraid of feeling lonely, go get another tribe of people. Inclusion is a two-way process.

We can celebrate being different, and really what I mean is being unique, being you, and living by your values and truth—not conforming to the normal, if that's not doing it for you. So if you challenge what needs challenging, step up to your purpose and lead yourself, can you imagine what life would look like from this place? We need to get people to step up and be included in the bigger picture. Many world class leaders, inventors, and thought leaders have had temporarily lonely lives, and as much as their brilliance gives us great comfort today, for those that had different ideas, pushing boundaries to see and do things that no one felt was possible, it was once very challenging and isolating. But they persevered and found inclusion in a small number of people who believed in them, and they succeeded in what they wanted.

We need this approach for as many in our population, and only then will we see leadership blossoming from more of us in a way that is congruent and fearless. The flip side would be people wanting to be the same, doing the same, thinking and feeling the same; and in time, their individualism, their uniqueness, and their inherent power and spirituality is lost. They traded it to hide amongst the masses, allowing others to dictate and even hypnotize them, and when they do try to voice their individualism, it gets cut down, hidden, and brushed under the carpet.

This isolation can be damaging. We have the right to be ourselves and uphold our culture, traditions, thoughts, and uniqueness, and like others, our human need is to give and receive love, no matter what area of life—family, work, community, or social enterprise. We need to be more inclusive and included. Racial tension and barriers will come down, and we will increase our abundance of humanity and diversity. We need to be unconditional in our response to unique ways, transcending cultural barriers and celebrating inclusivity for everyone. Our individual health and collective health are ONE. Our whole state of being this way will make changes to every cell in our bodies, its physiology, its genetics, and every way that outward science cannot change. It is only within us.

It is only with such inclusivity that we can feel that we belong to ourselves and then to others. If we only stay with people that keep us at the same level, we may feel great ease with them but also a little dead—like flat lining, and eventually dying. For real growth, if you want it enough, it is about finding someone who can challenge you for your own personal growth, so that you feel like you are about to take off from a cliff edge, and you feel real aliveness, where your heart beats like it's meant to, and you can feel it pumping like a well-toned muscle.

Many times during business networking meetings, I would come across people who would avoid me once they knew I was a lifestyle and health coach, because I was of no value to them. They did not know why, and I doubt they even reflected on it, but that avoidance was really interesting. I could see the discomfort in their body language, and many were just there to promote their businesses in such a narrow-minded way. Many were not really that authentic about their business success, and for those that were, they felt they did not need coaching, and that it's for the weak! You see, the problem is that if you have a good coach in front of you, DO NOT try and lie intentionally or unintentionally—we know. I know, and I knew. I don't judge. I don't have to, because the person spouting out superficial words is lying to themselves; they are, after all, their own judge and jury, or perhaps too ignorant, and perhaps even too self-obsessed. I saw and felt their ego in full swing. Can you position coaching in someone's life for their benefit then? No, I would have wasted my time and only irritated them. Did Steve Jobs' premature death not teach the world anything? Now, I know that this is also largely the British culture, the stiff upper lip and pride. What happens when you have a coach in front of you, and you don't stand in your own truth, is that the feeling of discomfort you feel is as if you are doing that to them, and people will naturally gravitate toward people who agree with what they are, and give out the exact mistruth.

Working with a coach that made me uncomfortable but loved me by holding me to account to be my best was the best thing I did for myself. What's the point of working with someone who makes you feel nice and comfortable? They just keep you at the same level. If you are choosing a coach, head over www.SanjayaPandit.com to "Choosing a Coach" to discover what type of coach you may find really helpful.

Do these people need coaching or some kind of mental brainwashing? Of course, they do. When they were asked why they would avoid us, the answers usually sat within this: "It was as if you were the mirror into my soul, which I did not want to admit to." I loved this answer then, and so much more now. It was a WOW. When asked what they wanted for their business, they said, "We want our business to grow." How is that even possible until you can learn and grow yourself? You need a coach that is going to challenge you appropriately and in service of your growth, not some coach who is hung up on being liked by clients and doesn't have the coaching range to work with.

The biggest limiting factor, and weakest link in any business, is the owner and then the people who run it, if you all do not grow in yourselves. Businesses, as we know, are happy to pay incredible money toward the harder skills training, and these courses are important; but without you implementing it, there is no point. It has to be you that needs to grow from within and take action, before your business can look like anything you dream about. For it to be healthy, you have to be healthy; after all, you are in charge. Sometimes stepping out and being bold is vital. Beware of what you are doing that is "safe in familiarity," especially if you are not getting the results or outcomes you want.

I want to be connected with people who challenge me the right way, teach me something new, and are living their dreams and purpose. Luckily, there have always been many in this tribe, including in a professional coaching network, so we get each other. When you are on this path, you will find us, and us you. Just by having the idea to write this book, I have met so many new people who are just as, or even more, ambitious as I am, and it is very exciting. When getting to know them, most have all used powerful and transformative personal coaches. The depth and breadth of their awareness and knowledge is truly remarkable.

Question for you:
"What makes you feel happy,
with a real sense of being included and belonging?"

Guiding principle:
"Without belonging and inclusion, you cannot breathe;
it's oxygen to your being, as long as it's authentic and sincere."

In Your Head

I am going to pick up on your internal dialogues in a bit more detail here, and look at it with you so that you are aware of the impact it has on you and people around you. Awareness of it will help allow you to seek for better engagement with your dialogue, so that you live a life free from sabotage, and instead focus on your greatness and your true ability and potential.

Our ability to think and feel through situations in our lives is our greatest asset, and yet it is under-utilised by many. What kind of life you desire is up to you, but you have a life and a purpose to it, even though you may not realise what it is—well, not fully anyway. If you know, that's fantastic, and if you don't, then it is surely in your best interest to live it in the most powerful way you can. It does not have to be a massive thing—with huge celebrity lights and lifestyle—it can be very simple as well, and it is important to qualify that for yourself. The most important thing, of whatever scale it is, is about being mindful to it, enjoying it with your heart and mind, and engaging and being in balance with it so that you can be in bliss. You may already have it and not even know it. For realisation and truth that is your life, training your mind to think in a way that allows for this life to be realised and sustained is fundamental.

We have thoughts that stem from our belief systems, memories, and experiences of earlier days. Our morals are influenced by the outside world. Our unique set and hierarchy of values also contribute to our thinking patterns. Putting it all together to train patterns of thought that are aligned for our best every day, is where it gets tricky for so many. It is like re-training a normal part of you, and that does take focus, energy, and commitment amongst other attributes. So imagine if we could all be more aware of the thoughts going through our heads, from much earlier on. Think of dog training for a few minutes, whether you have experienced ever training a new pup or a rescue dog. Puppies learn fast because they have a clean slate from which their foundation can grow; however, rescues dogs, who have troubled experiences, will be harder to train, and especially if they are older dogs, as some habits have been conditioned and have taken root. With new behaviour training, the best way is to repeat and reinforce, consistently, and then the dog's brain learns to automatically know the cues and commands, and acts out in the way that is desired. Again, it's about positive reinforcement, and dog training usually takes place with treats used for motivation and attention, from their owner who they love to please. We are NO different in that manner. Given the motivation, desire, and pleasure, we are the same in terms of positive reinforcement with rewards.

The power that lies within our minds and thoughts can dictate our emotions and therefore our behaviours; and what actions come about as a result, dictate our trajectory in life. Our thoughts become fixed in a cycle, and they go round and round, even without realising it. What we do know is the results, the evidence that we experience, and they can either be what we want or not what we want.

If the evidence is not what you desire, then you need to go back into your dominant thought patterns. We also know that some people think, think, and think, and actually very rarely put themselves into taking actionable steps, which mean outcomes also do not materialise. So you have to work out where you are at.

Thoughts of procrastination, as well as thoughts that sabotage you, can take root when you are not sure that the changes you want to make will ever work out, whether you really do deserve it, or will even succeed at it. Our greatness is the bit we are actually all scared of, and it is this that stops us from having what we want, because we think the change would have us living our lives so differently that we actually become stuck in the comforts of our smaller lives, and we learn to cope and justify it. All this is evidence of your thinking patterns—your self-talk. We are encouraged to fit in rather than stand out. As children, we are given the wrong trajectory and expectations of life. Girls are given the dream of happy-ever-after and finding their one love—their prince; and boys are given the script to be tough, strong, successful, and emotionless, before a princess will even kiss them. The world is such that unless you are in the right environment, no one likes a strong, capable, successful person with both heart and mind engaged; that is too perfect to be true, so people are wary of such people. If you are a woman like this, then it is even more challenging. As a woman, I can share plenty of times when I experienced this. When we try to step up, we get shot down, or the preference would be to hide— it's easier and less disruptive, and you don't feel so exposed. And that becomes what your head will tell you: that if you are nothing special, then more people will like you. So play down and play dumb, if you want to be liked. That is still the rhetoric of today.

But there is greatness in us all, and that's what we need to find, and until we do, we won't be able to rest—our calling, whatever that is, won't let us.

No matter how many material things you have, like money and nice cars, it is your higher purpose that's calling you, and some are nearer to it than others, because it becomes your happy way of life. I have met and witnessed so many people who, despite having a life of luxury, are still not joyous, and they actually have self-esteem issues and are unhealthy. They can't sit with themselves quietly, and they distract themselves from this feeling by keeping busy, busy, busy. Entrepreneurs are so performance driven that they forget to sit still— they can't—and they actually live very differently to their public persona. We all know countless sporting heroes and celebrities who are not "whole" when off screen or off stage, and they create unhealthy habits during this time. We have to watch that. No one can perform 100 percent of the time, so when you are resting, you only have yourself for company, and if you are not living your truth, can you imagine how uncomfortable that is? We want our hearts and minds to be free at this time with ourselves, and our conscience clear of any ill doing or ill being, so that it does not eat us up inside. So watch what your mind is saying to you. Is it the truth or a fabrication of it? Does it say what your heart tells you? Are they aligned? Is there a conflict?

We cannot live under an illusion or pretense; not for long anyway. It's cleaner and simpler to be authentic in every aspect. You can look in the mirror and feel good then, and nothing comes to haunt you ever. Being authentic is not easy because people around you don't know the value of it; they don't know it themselves so they may regard you as sly, arrogant, or too wise for your own good. The list is endless. They misinterpret you. Being yourself is worth it even if the road to your greatness is a lonely one for a short while. There are people like me who have walked it alone, so I know what it means to be in a tribe where people will cherish who you are and not what you are. By stepping up and out, you have the opportunity to clear that baggage that holds you down. You can rise up and meet other self-realised people, and the connection is magic. I have met some very successful entrepreneurs who can't look into anyone's eyes, and certainly not those of someone with a pure heart full of love.

The question you may have is whether I am talking about being on your path *and* being lonely. No, lonely is a different place to be. I am talking instead about being on your path, on purpose, to your higher self, which can sometimes mean that you have to leave people behind to find the truth, and let new people come into your life. You cannot connect to your inner wisdom amongst noise, so get away and be in tranquil settings.

I have been in business long enough to have had some really dark days, when everything I built for myself and my family was taken away, and I remember having to make changes in order to survive. Sometimes I had only 25 pence in my account, with children to feed and bills to pay; and creditors were chasing me for their money, and not believing me when I told them that I couldn't pay them, and then they would use their power to try and force unrealistic payments from me. However hard those times were, I kept my values and integrity, and I always strived for the best for myself and everyone. I still kept giving through my time, and I always found a way to feed myself and my children—little was better than nothing. They became better people for it. In fact, those experiences helped build great characters in all my four children, and built another important characteristic in me as if it was my final test: It rekindled my drive, and reawakened my purpose and contribution to the world. It gave me even more energy and a deep sense of freedom and happiness, which I cannot explain, but you may have felt it when despite all the circumstances against you, there is this gem of a spark, this deep sense of self-worth. It is a quiet, considerate voice, and that was my ally—my only ally. The fear that I once had, of having no money, just disappeared; that was liberating, and once again, I learnt something so valuable as I moved forward on my path.

I trust it like nothing else, and when I think back to those times, there are things that come to mind every time that are my greatest allies: my health; my mind being grateful and positive; my body that told me to rest, to play, and to keep eating well; and my spirit for its amazing faith and belief. This gift of my head, heart, and health allowed me to immerse myself in an experience without any distractions like pain or mental illness, and all my creativity and solutions came from within. My children and I were the only people that mattered, and how I have cultivated their upbringing to what I am teaching here in this book, is unique. They are my walking, talking, inspired inspirers.

I remember how my friends worried for me at these times of my lack of income and my increasing debts, and of possibly losing my house. They worried about how I would feed my dependents. They were so worried, and they gave advice all day long, which frankly, I switched off, because that felt like I was drowning, and despite me telling them that I felt fine and believed that it would all work out, and to have faith in this journey, they would come back and tell me that I was depressed, was not myself, that my energy was different, and that I was too solemn and was not talking about "taking over the world." They thought I was lost. My answer was that "I had found myself," and from that point, I had no fear or remorse, and all I saw was my greatness and the ability to nurture it for the next chapter of my life as my spirit ascents. For them and some others, the worry was genuine, but for many more, my focus gave no content to gossip from.

Knowing yourself and catching important transformational thoughts as life evolves through good and bad times, will protect you and guide you every step of the way. I am not saying that you should micromanage your thoughts and actions, but be aware of the patterns that change for the worse, or in my case for the better, even though my friends could not see me getting past this temporary situation. I could see myself getting past it, and I did; and by the way, they showed me lots of concern and advice, but not once did they actually offer to help me—funny, don't you think? I could and I did—that's all that ever mattered, and so did my children, the people that mattered. Sometimes people mean well, but it comes out all wrong, so understand and know yourself, and they won't make an imprint, with their fears or restrictive ways of thinking, on your mindset. It was also a time to assess those friendships, and I wonder and now laugh at how quiet they are when things go brilliantly for me, and the minute I say the opposite, they are all over me like a rash, with their guidance and advice, but very rarely will they actually do anything meaningful to help. I say let them be; they will eventually get it for themselves.

Instead, feed and surround yourself with people at your level of awareness; embrace their difference and their awareness about themselves, and connect in a much deeper, holistic way. It will be effortless if it is right, just as life is meant to be. Deeper social networks dictate how long and healthy and happy our lives will be. It is through having people like that around you that will contribute to how healthy, long, and joyous your life can be.

Becoming aware of your thoughts is the first step to your journey of greatness, ease, flow, and change. Do a comparative process when you are experiencing the magic in something happening to you, and also the opposite when things are not as well. There will be some obvious reasons and some very subtle reasons. The importance is to do the exercise in the first place if you really want to know. It is worthwhile!

Grab yourself a diary, where you can track your thought patterns as you go about your daily life, for about one or two months. This time frame allows for most that happens to you to happen, and you can really drill down into the awareness of your thoughts during this time. When you write down a thought or thoughts, also write down the corresponding emotion that comes with that thought, and see what you do or don't do.

Question for you:
"What are your most dominant thoughts daily,
and how do you generally feel when you think them?"

Guiding principle:
"If you master your mind, you will master your life,
and anything you desire for the greater good is possible then."

Generations of Learning – Right or Wrong?

Who we are and what we become is learnt from the people we spend the most time with, and if you think back to your childhood, it was most likely your parents, grandparents, and brothers and sisters; and some of us had nannies or child minders, teachers, and perhaps neighbours that were just as influential.

If you then take every individual you have known, and think about their influence on you, and then think of their own sphere of influence when they were children, and so on and so on, you can start to understand the magnitude of what gets passed about, around, and up and down. So you actually have generations of people and learning in your head, and with that, you also have learnt information that seems consistent with generations of teaching, learning, and influence.

However, each of us has the capability of interrupting patterns of learning, behaviours, thoughts, and mindsets at any time once we become aware of thought patterns, and this can be good or bad. There are many that had troubled childhoods, who through their change in thinking, gave themselves the drive to aspire to better ways, and that's all it takes; but the road can be challenging, with ups and downs. Accept that; don't fight it, and you will get through. With every challenge, it tests your commitment and true desire.

Challenges can, in the short term, cause trouble in relationships. Remember when you tried to change something that had been in the family for a lifetime, and you experienced an unsupportive point of view? All that it is, is new information, which takes time to process; and in relationships, what one does affects another in ways that cannot be predicted, but it does not mean your relationship is failing just because you don't see eye to eye at times.

Remember, we all like to be in our comfort zones—the places where we are familiar with practiced ways and predictable outcomes.

There can be discomfort when we embark on something new, and people start expressing their opinions about how you cannot do this or that, and why you should do it this way. Some will challenge who you are and why you just can't do it; the once "loved one" can become your "demon," pointing out everything that stands in your way. Does that fear belong to you or them? What can it be?

There will be times that you will feel discomfort or be defensive on some of the discussion points in this book, because it may not relate to your experience, or you may be stuck in a place where you think you know it all, and I may have challenged you to think of your health outcomes or a way of life in a different way. The content and my ideas are not meant to be enforced; they are just meant to open you up to other perspectives of equal value.

When the change you seek has a method to get to where you want it to be, and you start implementing it into your life, then people will notice. Not all will want the best for you, so remember that. It is a little like sticking your head above water, where you get seen and you become a target to be shot down because something about you is different. And although your desire is sincere and does not involve stepping on anyone's shoes, you are nevertheless regarded as a threat, to be shot down before your wings get stronger. I have experienced this, and I have to say that this type of negativity is about fear in others, and again, a lack of their self-awareness. Our education and upbringing do not allow for curiosity because that "killed the cat!"

Even your loved ones, who you would just expect to support you no matter what, can sabotage you, especially if it affects them in some way, because they fear that the relationship will be changed for the worst—yes, an assumption made from a stuck perspective—which is terrible for people who hate any kind of change! Examples of changes could be when entering into a new relationship after a divorce; or a change of lifestyle that demands losing excess weight, which may get you looking rather more attractive again, and confident; or changing your career and thus meeting new people.

It happens, but you can think and behave better; talk it through and reassure the ones making the fuss around you. Most, however, go about it the wrong way. They try hard to change people's minds by arguing and chasing them to come round to their way of thinking—but stop right there; you can only change yourself! They will come round, so put all that energy into your mission, and when they are ready to listen and shift their perspectives, they will return in a way that you can have an adult conversation.

So, how can we get support and put an end to the generation of voices, saboteurs, and fearful committees that prefer to stay in one place, and even more so, keep you in the same old place?

Well, mostly, it is about communication, expression, and reassurance; and the first rule is to not let anyone get in your way once you have made a decision that feels right. Some relationships will be challenged, and you may make the decision to part; and some relationships will get closer—hooray! These are the people you want around you in the present because they will support you during both the good and bad times, unconditionally. Remember, sometimes a loved one's reaction is not to support, but they do come round eventually, so give them the space to let them process the impact of your change on them. Such news makes them engage their primal brain, which is all about familiarity, safety, and comfort. Anything that challenges that gets rejected. If the foundation of attachment with them is healthy and thriving, it will work out in the end.

You may just be the person that inspires change in others, and that's all you can do. Change yourself and let that be a catalyst for others if they want it. You become an inspiration to them. So, no matter how difficult, or what the voices in your head are saying that are negative and unhelpful, don't give in. Focus on what you want every day until you have it. It is therefore really crucial to get the basics right, from the start. Without change, we would be doomed, because our need for challenge and correct stimulation would not be met in our lifetime—remember the need for structure, as our brains need it, and from an emotional point of view, we need it just as we do air to breathe. It's that basic. It is life-giving.

What are the patterns of learning you have in your life? I say "patterns" because we are looking for repetitions; the consistency reinforces and embeds it into our lives, whatever the quality. You know sayings like, "Money comes to us hard," "We can't be rich like them," and "We are big boned in our family, so we can't be thin."

Such statements are definite and absolute, and our brains believe that they cannot be changed. The worst thing is that we are not even aware of them, but we can notice this from our unhelpful behaviours that tell us what can be deeply embedded in our minds. As long as you become more aware of them, they can be changed. You will feel and act differently, which is more consistent with your new thoughts. So when you hear a thought that is self-limiting and is no longer true or serving the best in you, and it comes from someone in your present or past sphere of influence, write it down or make a mental note; become aware of the associated feeling and actions involved, and then interrupt the pattern by consciously thinking about something better. Think of important aspects of life you once wanted and still don't have, and become aware of the battles you have in your head about certain things going on for you—that intel needs to be heard by you.

These are some more questions to really get curious about on these limiting thoughts from your unforgiving committee. How did these thoughts and beliefs best serve you in the past? Did they? What about today? What would happen if you continue listening to these unhelpful statements and voices? What's the corresponding emotion with this awareness? What's that telling you?

Imagine what you can offer to yourself and the people who you love when you are more self-aware, and any changes you want to make come from this place of knowing yourself. What impact will that have on you and others that have you in their lives? I am sure that you have heard about the ripple effect. It starts with a central position, a central force and energy—YOU!

I have worked with people of all ages and experiences, and there has been such a variation in their upbringing; and at times, some became so confused with who and what they were. Their minds ruled them, or rather other's influence ruled them! Life was a struggle for them, but what transpired was a rebirth of the mind when they took action to discover themselves. It is a bold step and, for many, it is full of fear of the unknown. But when they did, it was like they pulled the cord on their computer and rebooted it again, with fresh updated ideas and ways of living. Suddenly, life at source was injected back, and hope filled them up. They were transported to a truly transformational resonant place, and from this place—again, with some help from me and my coaching—they started putting pieces together in a more functional, authentic way. They found themselves and stopped living someone else's life. They took ownership and responsibility, and accepted that they could reboot at any time, because what happened afterwards was beautiful to watch and be part of. That's the learning taking place at a deeper, more resonant level.

Can we all have this? Yes! Yes! Yes!

It is an individual's choice, but the world's problems cannot be solved if we remain ignorant of ourselves and our worth. If we are each of us at our best, optimal in every way, then we also give out our best. It is a win-win!

Question for you:
"What is your thought right now?
What's the full impact of it as you become aware of it?"

Guiding principle:
"Learn to get good and skilled at understanding your thoughts and all their consequences—that means to evaluate their associated emotions in you, and also your actions or inactions."

But Who Wins Sometimes? Who's Talking?

When you get to that kind of awareness, and suddenly you are so empowered to make some changes to be your best and to live your dream life, what also wakes up is the saboteur: "Who do you think you are?" It wakes up like a sleeping virus and is ready to disrupt, because the bigger the change, and the bigger the challenge, the bigger the saboteur. It's like the "bigness" of your dream just fed it, and it becomes the monster of doom and gloom, trying every which way to derail you, joining forces with the generations of saboteur voices from within; and what you get is a battle of wills, disharmony, dissonance, and the feeling of overwhelm and heaviness, pulling you backwards and forwards, turning you and your life upside down, inwards and backwards. Have you experienced anything like this?

If you have, you will know exactly what I am talking about, and it may vary in magnitude and depth, but it is similar and the outcome it wants is the same: to stop you. It wants to bring you to a dead-end, where it is easier to go back to where you came from. It is exhausting, is it not?

Swimming against this current, keeping what you want in focus—your goal, your dream, your mission—is very hard, and it takes a lot of active energy, but swim against it you must, because there is your empowerment and success. Could you do this without your health being the best? Can you understand the psychology of health here, and also your physical form, which needs to be at its best because, otherwise, the saboteur will know where you are weak—in mindset, in spirit, or in your body. People have reported chest pains when there was no problem with their heart; it's a psychosomatic pain, but one that can scare you enough that you stop going forward on your new path anyway.

The difficulty of striving for what you want is the number one reason why so many people give up on something they want so badly! They lose hope. Some never get started because they don't want to experience this sort of difficulty or hard work. Just as inspiring as it is to share the struggle of getting there, for some, this knowledge can also be disempowering; so people like me, speakers, authors, and coaches, have a responsibility to share wisdom and experience to empower the majority. You know the saying: "Something worthwhile is never easy." Change is difficult, and human change even more so. Stop allowing stubborn core beliefs and these voices to run your life.

What you want to decide on is what impact your chatter has on your life, and what to change for the better. This is, in most cases, the stumbling block, because it's not known fully, so making half measures and unrealistic changes is the wrong focus, and it is where the results are not what you would expect. So let's gain some clarity and make decisions as to how it's going to be. For health and wellbeing, I picture blocks that keep you stuck, where you can see forward but you can't physically get past them. You become stuck there. Listen to any suggestions that come from awareness that they are not aligned to your goals on health and wellbeing, but work out whether it is your best self talking to you or your demon in a kinder disguise. Don't take any action that reinforces the beliefs you are trying to change.

Question for you:
"Don't you think it may be a good idea to stop listening to those voices of doom? They have surely overstayed their welcome."

Guiding principle:
"Listen to your loving adult. You are the captain of your ship and you are the master, so listen to that inner guidance and start rising to your inherent potential."

Why Do We Do What We Know Is Bad for Us?

Can you answer this for yourself or for people that you know? Does it make sense? If it was so simple, then we would not smoke, or take medication, drugs, or alcohol, or get stressed, overeat, or pick bad foods to feed ourselves, and diabetics would stop sneaking those chocolates—or would they?

There is no simple answer when it comes to us humans and our ways, especially when we convince ourselves that "one more won't hurt," when we know it does; or we say things like, "Well, it's only a little cheat," or "We only live once, so we may as well enjoy it."

Adding to this unhelpful internal dialogue is when we take a good look around us, at people, places, eateries, supermarkets, and the media. So many of the messages from them contribute to our detriment because we cannot manage ourselves in this environment; it gives us so much temptation that we have become abusive to ourselves through the choices we are making daily. We chase happy, social acceptance; fun; and superficial belonging and inclusion. It is the developing landscape that concerns me because it is harder to stay well and do the things that we are meant to do by being our true selves. The problem is, we end up with an extreme way of thinking, and we go from one end of the spectrum to another. Those who are totally evangelical, and almost paranoid, would never stray off their path to the other side of the spectrum, where people just don't give a damn about anything—they excessively smoke, overeat, and drink until they recognise that time is up and they have just been denied 10 years of their life span. What really goes on for such people? What are they trying to prove to themselves and others? I don't think they even know, because it's just not rational.

I have worked with a group of people who generally feel so empty that they need to keep full with food and drink. Likewise, yo-yo dieters swing from one base to another, each time getting further and further from balance and health. We are only required to live in a balanced way, and finding balance is the game of life. Balance is your ultimate goal. It is achievable and does not require extreme measures, even though out of balance can be extreme.

The difficulty is this; let me give you an example of a conversation I was a witness to at an airport, when we were all waiting to board a plane back to the UK. The group beside me comprised of three people—two men and a woman—and it seemed that they were waiting for a fourth person, a lady who they spoke about in a joyful, fun way. It seemed that she had missed her flight many times before, and they were asking each other whether she was even awake, and then remarked that they would not be surprised if she missed the flight. In the ten minutes, I witnessed them talking quite loudly about her, and not once did they call her by her real name. Instead, I learnt about her from the labels and identity they had created for her—"the 100-a-day fag queen," and the "drunk shag diva," amongst other sayings, and these were her so-called work colleagues! I became really uncomfortable and tried to stop myself from listening in, but I was hooked, and they were so loud that, to be honest, I was not the only one subjected to this conversation.

Then, after about 15 minutes of her ridicule in her absence, I noticed a woman walking toward us, and she looked normal. She joined them and had no idea of the gossip-type conversation about her a few minutes back, where she was the subject of their entertainment. They then started questioning her as colleagues bantered, speaking to her and asking questions on if she had been stopped at security, or if she had managed to raid the duty-free of all its cigarettes. They voiced their observation that she was walking remarkably straight for having drunk too much last night. She, of course, as expected, delighted in all the attention she was getting, and she often laughed at herself. On the surface, it was all a little banter and taking the mick, and having fun, but I felt that there was a serious undertone. I was offended for her, so why was she not—or was she, and pretended to not be?

If you now think back to the points made earlier about attention and inclusion, how can someone allow others to have a laugh on them? This type of person would find it incredibly challenging to change; imagine if she turned up at the next conference squeaky clean, no cigarettes, and no alcohol, and instead holding a bottle of green juice. What would the three colleagues say then? They would gossip there too!

Do you think they may feel really uncomfortable and awkward in her company, if she no longer laughed at herself in such a demeaning way? Yes, absolutely, guaranteed. It's an isolating place, at least for a while, and it is because of this that so many do not venture forth any more than they have to. They don't complete their change process; they give up, give in, or sabotage through their thoughts.

What would it have taken for one of them to say: "Stop this; you are better than people laughing at you and ridiculing you, and what is more, it's not healthy to drink and smoke so much—what's going on? If you don't stop this, you could get very ill and possibly die before your time." Could you have that conversation with her? Can you be courageous and bold enough to hold out on what is her best version of herself?

This is what I am talking about: the value of your health, your life, and your best potential, and then every other living being. In the UK especially, we have a real reputation for a drunken binge culture—it is terrible! It's wrapped up in being part of something, where to be a laugh is better; it provides a great feeling to you, and entertainment to others, and you become everyone's friend, and the justification to be labelled or ridiculed for your ways is done. The problem is that it starts quite early on. Just observe teenagers of today in the UK, and now the sad fact of where its prevalence was not as high in my culture; it is becoming that way albeit hidden at times from strict parents who think of their children as squeaky clean. I do some silly things sometimes to let my hair down, but it's neither dangerous to me nor to others, and I certainly don't engage in activities that make me a regular laughing stock, and on which my entire reputation is built. Yes, I have worn funny things that make people laugh, for a charity event; but the next day, I go back to the usual, with a fond memory of the laugh we all had, and a memory created that connected us in that comical moment. I don't have an empty void to fill with food or alcohol, or with habits that are plain unhealthy.

This lady's colleagues do not want the best for her but are happy to ridicule her because she allows it. Is that valuing herself, or is she so confident that she doesn't care what people think? Maybe I need to chill out and not take it so seriously, but I could not help but feel bad for her, and wanted to tell her colleagues to stop it, and ask them if they would say those things to her face. Maybe part of me wanted to help her get help so that she could get away from that auto destruct path she may be on. Would those same colleagues be there for her in her hour of need, perhaps as gratitude for the hours of entertainment she provided for them? Or would they just state that she brought that on herself? Could they even once look to see what responsibility they played in this? No one likes to take the blame and be responsible, but instead it's easier to be cowardly and pretend that nothing is wrong than stand up for yourself or for someone else, because it's harder to be in that place.

If you witness yourself or anyone else in self-destruct mode, even while having fun, pull yourself or them out of it, no matter how hard it is. Your health and life will be indebted to you, and your relationship with yourself and with them will be stronger; much stronger, and if not, let them go.

Even through a long shot, if they said something but she did not do anything else, then she was not ready to change and live her truth. Would you let someone talk about you in a negative light, ridiculing you? And would you remain friends with them?

You know that familiarity of your comfort zone, even when things are not good as a result, but the difference between that and changing something is scary and not easy; so what happens is that we choose the easy option and justify reasons for this. It has to make sense, so we go through our catalogue of every possible incident and scenario so that it sounds rational and chosen. We sabotage what we also know is the one good way. What you may not realise in that moment is the years of feeling guilty or letting yourself down, doing things you KNOW are bad for you. You can end up carrying this around with you for years, and for some of you, to your last day on earth.

Can you imagine the serious damage such emotions can have on your long-term health, or when trying to change your health for the better? I know people who have made themselves sick because of it, yet they are blind to understand that it was that unhelpful choice in that moment that gave them the permission to do it again and again and again, until that became their identity; and the all-knowing wisdom that they once had, of what is right, got buried deep down.

This lady who not once was addressed by her real name, may have pointed her finger of blame at her heavy schedule of travel, temptations of booze and cigarettes, or even the colleagues that she entertained and who encouraged her bad habits by paying attention to them in a joking way; but one day, I hope she will find that her gift of life and its meaning and importance rises, and she begins her journey of self-discovery.

It is always easier to blame something or someone at the start of self-discovery and enlightenment; but point your finger at something, and see how many fingers point back at you. It is always about you; it always starts with you, so instead of making excuses, and complaining and thinking that your mistakes are about someone else or something else, always remember the message that is in both of your hands: When you point a finger, you have three pointing at YOU!

It is quite incredible that our fingers on our hand are built in such a way that the mechanics also give us signs in this regard. We need to take responsibility for our choices, and wherever possible, equip ourselves with awareness, and then act on the information we realise. Taking responsibility is the only way to progress, and it can change your thinking completely, inspire you to problem solve, and create a way of life that you truly deserve.

Question for you:
"What are you hard wired to do or be that is bad for your health?"

Guiding principle:
"Your greatest attribute is to value yourself highly
and always, whilst staying humble, kind, generous,
and grateful to every living being."

Stubborn Learnt Habits

A habit is something you have learnt, reinforced, and then repeated, which then supports it as a habit. It becomes stubborn because you have a stubborn or a matter-of-fact, absolute core belief attached to this habit. Any desire to change this habit feels difficult and awkward, and the emotional response to the change can be enough of a discomfort, so the natural state is to recoil back to this habit, as this feels more conditionally natural now.

To undo habits that are stubborn, it will take a good measure of focus, not just on the physical interruption but also in the mind. If you do not believe that what you are changing is of benefit to you, you won't have the motivation. Without your own motivation, you cannot action anything toward such change, and will instead recoil soon after and not finish what you started. You may be able to recollect that getting into bad habits did not take as much effort as it does to regain the "before." Let's face it, most bad habits are comforting: biting nails, eating sugar and candy, talking yourself out of effort and exercise. There are 100s of habits that do not serve us, and the way we think of them also needs effort to change.

What stubborn and unhelpful habits do you have? Which three habits can you focus on to change? Which have you tried changing? What happened, and where are you now with them? If you have been successful in changing one thing, you have the skills to change another, even if it is a different habit. That's all you have to know. It comes down to belief and understanding and patience. You must know that time and consistency are your additional allies in unlearning stubborn, unhelpful habits.

So let's get really clear on what such habits you have, and I am asking you to focus on the three most impactful ones. Take a piece of paper and write down all the habits being practiced at the moment, which you know are not very helpful for your health and wellness. What emotions and statements or ways of thinking go with them? You can specify them against areas of your life, or habits that you have tried to change in the past but returned to quickly. Once you have written as much down as you can become aware of, ask someone that you live with to add to what they see as your bad habits, which they are concerned with for your health. This is because we are often blind to our most stubborn habits. We dismiss them and have a way of not really being aware of them. It's that automatic process, and in our justification to keep the change at bay, we discount the serious impact of them. A tip would be to include a habit that is relatively easier in your view to break out of. You will notice that there are different degrees of ease and difficulty for some of your habits, so don't go straight in. In this first instance, and when choosing three hard habits that you want to break, just include one that gives you an easier win.

Then qualify each habit in terms of what it is and how it is serving you today. What is outdated about it, and whose habit is it really? Where did you learn it?

Then take the 3 habits, if you have them from areas across the range of your life, and write them down on the left-hand side of the paper. On the right-hand side, write down its replacement habit. It could be a habit that someone has that inspires you and may be really helpful— you know, like when you hear yourself saying, "I wish I could do that," while you observe this person!

I want you to learn this method of breaking habits, and then this can be applied to the tougher ones later.

A habit that I wanted to create when I became self-employed, was getting up a little earlier. I think I justified the lie-ins because I lost so much sleep during years of child rearing. I don't know to this day how I coped, and I also worked late into the evening but had to get up for the school run, so there was no getting away from the ritual for years. I did find that getting up earlier, by at least half an hour, gave me the peace of mind to look after myself instead of being thrusted into child care the minute I woke, because that resulted in me missing out or multi-tasking, or hurrying up on my things and rushing through the quality of my standards. It also meant that I could get the business strategy end of my business progressing nicely within the first 90 minutes of my day, after which I could see to customers, business support, administrative duties, and staffing. I could also rest again before the onslaught of client workshops began at 4:30 p.m. till late.

In the UK, during winter, this is really not easy because it is so dark; my body clock was telling me to prepare to sleep and not to rise until much later. At 5:30 a.m., it is really too dark here, so I compromised and agreed that 6:15 a.m. would be good to have a go at, even at weekends. It was tough, and I don't like alarms, so I had to train my mind to naturally wake up; and for a long time, my chatterbox suggested snoozing, but I persevered by having something wonderful to wake up to, like a ritual. So my one hour before all the children were up for school, was my time to meditate and spend a few minutes, after having my tea, out in the cold at sunrise, which for me connects me to nature and just refreshes me. I know it is not for everyone, but for me, getting that little bit of fresh air was like heaven and so very refreshing. I did this for 30 days and promised myself an evaluation at the end. It worked out so well that I carried on for a further 30 days, and it has now been a few years since I started this for myself. It is now a habit but not so inflexible that I am a slave to it.

I test it from time to time by having a lie-in—for me, that's like 8, and at the latest, 9 a.m. I can't do that anymore, and not with ease—I guess I don't want to either—I think it is a waste of my day and it makes me feel lethargic, and it is annoying when I have to rush things again. It is just not worth it. I like grounding myself so that I am at peace with myself. The important thing to learn about making new better habits is to associate them with something rewarding and beneficial that is NOT a contradiction. So, for example, if you are creating better ways of eating healthier foods, don't reward yourself with a binge-eat down at the local Chinese. Do that a few times because you think that you are way too far into your new habits of eating healthier, and I promise you that the claw back will be compelling. Instead, reward yourself with something different.

Question for you:
"What are the stubborn habits you want to do without?"

Guiding principle:
"Breaking stubborn habits that impact your health
in a negative way is one of the best things you can do."

Chapter principle:
"Your basic need for food and water and environment is tied in with basic psychological needs. Many go at improving health without these principles in place, and that is why it is difficult to attain health in a way that is sustainable. You may all have the physical basics, like food and water, in abundance, but the way you are with yourself and the people you have in your life also says a lot. First know yourself before you know anyone else."

Healthy Foundations – Getting Your Health Where It Belongs

Chapter 5
The Start

Back to Basics

When it comes to health and wellbeing, we are usually good at knowing what is needed. The problem is not what we know but doing it—actually implementing that knowledge and taking the first step, getting started and then continuing it, whatever that is and whatever it takes, consistently. But what happens instead? We procrastinate, and we find that we are not doing what we need to; one way of hiding our inaction is to seek more knowledge from as many places and people as possible. If that information or knowledge budges you further toward action, then great. Many, however, don't move forward; instead, they are more confused, and they freeze with indecision, and then that's not going to be good. Many look for the perfect formula before they even test the landscape of true health. Let me tell you, there is no perfect formula, but there is a formula that can kick-start your journey, and a formula that is bespoke and can evolve with you and for you.

Believe me, I have been with procrastination with health many times and kept coming back full circle. I again went through this process when I decided that I wanted to write a book and share my wisdom on true optimal health. It was a bizarre mix of excitement, empowerment, and then a fear of failure, and of disappointment of being judged. I felt and thought that I may not be quite good enough. Sometimes I felt like I was almost ready and was standing on the edge, and then I took a step back; and it went on like that for a number of years until I literally had to close my eyes and press a button to get the script to my publisher and his team. I had to remind myself what mission I was on and what a wonderful opportunity it was that was given to me through my experiences and solutions that can help others. This deal is so big, yet I still allowed myself to become little again, caving in. I went inside my head again and listened to false information about myself and my book, and for a few years, that got in my way. There were other legitimate reasons of course, but that's for another time. If I had not taken the step to get away from my own critique, you would not be reading this right now, so I am happy for us both.

Instead, let me say this to you: You know enough to get started, and what you need to learn will show up along the way; and any true and gifted lessons to learn will keep showing up repeatedly, and will not leave you alone until you learn whatever the lesson is trying to teach you! What is important is where and what we are in our understanding and knowledge of what we already know of ourselves, right here and right now, so work with that.

I love learning and tweaking my knowledge, updating it wherever and whenever needed. For that, I have an open mind. We need to challenge beliefs of our own and that of others, especially if they negatively impact lives. Our human duty to ourselves is to learn and to grow, and to stay healthy whilst doing it. We were not created to destroy ourselves, so it's helpful to check what is contributing to your health, and whether it is positive or negative. I also know that too much information can leave us so lost that in the process, we also lose our clarity and our own guiding intuition and intellect.

When we don't put our good knowledge and wisdom to use, and instead open ourselves to unreasonable influence and scam, we suffer. We need to listen wholeheartedly, trust ourselves with qualified information, and have the paradigm shift, knowing that we are good enough, and good at learning new skills and solving any problems that occur from time to time. If health is a problem for you, it doesn't have to be, but there are certain things you need by your side to restore it and get it on the right path.

One of the biggest deals of our time is prescription medicine, and yet so many people are ignorant of the fact that there seems to be an increase in their side effects, and even death. People simply are not able to tolerate these side effects, and if you are on a cocktail of medications, this can cause lasting complications. Drugs can interact with the food we eat and the lifestyles we lead, causing detriment and suffering. The problem is that we label health disorders and disease without looking at the full picture for every individual, and so the general prescribing methods become a "hit and miss." Whereas I have known people to gain massive benefit from prescription drugs, we are coming to the knowledge and truth that many pharma drugs being given to manage patients are unnecessary and can deteriorate overall health. For many of today's lifestyle diseases, it is unnecessary to prescribe pharmaceutical drugs. In fact, many argue that part of the management of disease in the past with such drugs has made health worse. I know what medicine did for me whilst treating my diabetes, and the effects were not good; and with consultation with my doctor, I decided to stop them. That may not be for everyone, and it is important to seek medical guidance from your doctor as we are all different; however, I know that lifestyle measures are even more effective for me than any drug could be.

It is time that the medical community give their patients a choice as to which way best serves their health, and definitely a change in the dinosaur age of the medical community having an allegiance only to the pharmaceutical community, by also partnering with lifestyle functional holistic practitioners and health coaches to give the patient informed choice as to the best and most individual way to treat and manage disease. Until then, doctors will be regarded as highly paid pharmacy distributors, and this image of them is catching on fast.

There is tremendous value to this highly skilled professional network of intelligent people, and it is time that they returned to their true desire, despite being handcuffed by the system. Surely, it is good to restore the medical community back to its proper collective wisdom, an educational institution looking for answers and providing solutions based on a transparent and effective relationship with each patient.

Is it that even the health service has fallen foul to marketing tricks? After all, the definition of marketing is that it solves a problem and fits a need, so why are our doctors not fitting a need: a desire for health and wellness. Perhaps if that was the case, then more people would take account of their illness and instead go and seek the proper help at the right time. So many of us are in denial of illness, and of the signs and symptoms that suggest something may be wrong. It is easier to ignore it until you can't! Perhaps that may also be contributed to the disconnection that is apparent among individual doctors. They are no longer of value, with people waiting for over an hour, only to tell them something just to gain medicine, because people in this category are actually more motivated to quick fixes. So we cannot really blame doctors, can we? We also need to blame ourselves for driving the chaos that is now unleashed with pharma drugs and their inappropriate use today. We want to be fixed, and they want to fix us quickly; I mean, not a lot can be done in 10 minutes, apart from a quick overview of symptoms, and then a prescription given, and to be told that if that doesn't work, then to come back—and you are not allowed to talk about anything else that is going on for you in your health. One appointment slot for one thing. How can that ever be a practice that tries to find the root cause and what is causing the symptom? It is highly "text book," putting you in boxes rather than looking at the whole picture.

We become sucked into quick fixes, thinking it will give us this and that, when actually it worsens it for us. If the root cause is not dealt with, it's symptoms and the way they show up will continue, each one and each time getting louder and more urgent—that's the body's way of telling you TO LISTEN! So we have to get better on knowing our bodies, understanding them better and appreciating them greatly. Until we can understand what value good health is, and how to protect it, we will not resolve anything, because we can run to the doctors and get creams and potions. This is the point of this book, teaching each other the value of health and that health is not just about eating right and exercising, because many that do are still just as sick, which means there are other important factors being dismissed. We all know, when someone comes to a near death experience, and when they recover by fighting for their life, how they understand what living was all about. It's when you don't have something that you understand the value of it. It's like another chance for them. They think it is a miracle and then take note; they suddenly become evangelical and very serious, continuing their newfound passion and purpose by writing books on it, creating charities for it, and talking about it. Why do we need to be near untimely death before we really understand health and its gifts? Some don't make it—they die—it's simply too late.

Some people—many people, I dare say—will continue day to day, taking no responsibility for their health, and we have to respect that this is their choice. People with meaning and purpose to their lives will not do that—they will take responsibility. Where are you? Or what are you waiting for?

I find it so interesting that people I have known over the years would do anything to raise money for cancer research—to show the world a degree of nobility in them, right? But then behind the scenes, the same lot don't value their own health. Straight after the event, say a fun run or something, they go straight home to pop open a bottle of wine and eat excessively as a reward. They smoke, and they only exercise when they have a fun run to get through; then it stops, and then they yo–yo back to their unhealthy lifestyle.

It's almost as if they become detached from what they are seen to be doing and what they *actually* do, and there is a degree of shame involved here because, let's face it, you would not want to show that to the world, but doing something noble may correct the pretense. The truth is that if they continue that way, there will be someone else raising funds for a fun run, in their name. There is a lack of integrity and congruency here, which I think needs addressing. It's actually a lot of hard work to lead a double life in anything. Don't; it's not necessary. I wish cancer charities would stop promoting food fundraisers, especially cake when we have an obesity epidemic, and that it is processed refined sugar and all its forms that can increase the risk of certain cancers anyway. It's hypocrisy, and again, not thought through. Yes, cake brings people together, and it's easier to raise funds on something as generic and inexpensive as cake that people like, but let's take some responsibility here. When we have such a huge mass of the population that is overweight or obese, they will be taking part in eating those cakes, and it won't just be one slither of a slice—it will be substantial pieces, and it doesn't stop there. They feel bad, so they eat more; they are scared of getting cancer, so they eat more—it becomes a self-fulfilling prophecy.

So, when you finally make a decision as to how you want to live your life, then you will attract things to make it easier for you to live exactly that way, and health and wellness will be your foundation on which to build.

Most people are stuck in the past and too much into the future, without being in the present. That in itself is a disease. Let us all concentrate on the present; it allows all the universal laws to work with you and for you.

Going back to basics is crucial. We have learned to overcomplicate health in our lives and those of others. If I were to say that going back to basics is THE first step in this process of changing the health paradigm for you, what would going back to basics mean to you? What would be the value of it? When and how can you start? Back to basics, in my view, is to simplify health and reset it with proven ways, using our all-important boundaries and discipline to guide us. Back to basics does not mean giving up on anything that you have grown to love; it's more about managing and moderating, and using the kinds of information that is genuine and validated in theory and in practice and in technology, yet embracing all the wisdom that comes from the past—the way our elders tried to educate us with their tried, tested, and practiced wisdom.

It makes so much sense to me because I am of the generation that can embrace the two worlds—the past 45 years and the present—and when I reflect on the changes that are happening, and the way that people live now, I have to say that my old fashioned values and wisdom come to the top and guide me more today than any new information, or rather misinformation, of today. The downside is that when I share this with my children, they obviously view me as some dinosaur, because they just cannot relate, and so I feel inspired to keep sharing things with them because it will have an effect eventually. It is a way of keeping them in touch with my childhood and the ways of before, that in my view have a great value for their lives today. My job would be to get them to experience some of that whilst keeping what they like and know today—that means phones, social media, and the different way they develop friendships and maintain friendships. I don't think they have ever written an actual handwritten letter to a friend or received one—it is all done on Instagram or Snapchat. That there poses a problem because they are constantly in touch with each other; there is no break, and I think that some distance from friends, no matter how close, every now and again, is healthier. I can reconnect with my earlier days so well, and that is the way I ground myself, and teach my children things from my past that are very much the answer to the present and future.

So how about spending some time to understand and fully acknowledge some basics in your life that have a dramatic effect on your daily life, and give your health really positive results. How do these things impact parts of your life that are important?

With a blank piece of paper, write them all down, and think about what basics are important for you to contribute to sustaining and improving your health and those of your loved ones. "Big up" health. Don't just think of a run or eating more vegetables; what about mind health, emotional, and spiritual health—whole health as I call it? If you do one thing, yes, it has been shown to impact another part of health, but not always, so being mindful of all these components so that they get the attention, is vital.

Write down all the things you are aware of that are detrimental to you, and you never quite get around to implementing or changing something about it; it stays more as a wish rather than an action you can take. What needs to happen to you for it to be implemented?

What is it you are already doing that is serving your health, and how can you include new ways and insight to give you a much more holistic picture of your health and lifestyle as you move forward?

Think also about balance. All our bodily systems are designed to balance, and they work very hard to keep it as near to that as possible—a form of homeostasis. We need to listen so that when our bodies give us intelligence or feedback when things are not right, we need to become skilled at listening to this with all our attention. Signs such as aches and pains, chronic illness, lower immunity function, digestive problems, headaches, and so on are all part of the mix for deteriorating lifestyle health and an imbalance. Watch that head of yours, and put any skeptical thoughts or thoughts of sabotage to one side whilst you do this part! We don't need it to fool you into thinking, "Be brave, be strong," as this can damage the natural calling for balance within your body and mind. Men especially, please take note here! It's about learning to listen, sitting still, and hearing yourself intuitively understand yourself and what is important and the way forward. We look for our answers outside of us when actually there is only one person that knows you so intimately: you yourself—so trust yourself with all your heart.

Knowing what you know does not always stop you from doing unhelpful things. This is where procrastination rears its ugly head, and unhelpful thoughts define our actions or inactions: What don't you know about nutrition really? What don't you know about how to exercise your body? What don't you know about sleeping and restful times? What don't you know about having fun and laughing? I know there is already knowledge and experience there for you. We just need to take action in the right direction, and start again from the beginning if we have to, and align this with the bigger vision of your life and your higher self. It is all connected. So start today, this minute!

Before Alice came to me for coaching, she told me how she sought help from nutritionists and personal trainers, who did help her to a degree, but her issues were still there, and any weight or food regimes she was introduced to, she found very difficult to sustain, even though it was really simple. She realised after plunging vast amounts of money into seeking help, that she was not ready, and that was what actually stopped her from understanding her motives and knowing herself.

She learned that she knew everything she thought she needed, and she just was unconsciously testing their expertise. She was asking another expert to tell her about herself, right?!

She lived by testing them, to prove something to herself, and to justify that she was half-heartedly dealing with herself, and that maybe this one would fix her for good; but she knew they were no better than some doctors who just gave her symptomatic relief and never really dealt with the real issues. They did not know how to! She expected everyone else to motivate her and sort her out. This carried on for 6 years of her life, and she poured almost £35,000 into finding solutions, but she went about it the wrong way. She already knew that the answers were within herself. Then she spent a little more to be coached by me. She set about working with me, and with my unique skills and no-nonsense approach, it gave her the clarity and solutions that she had wanted for so long. I would much rather she had paid herself £35,000 for those 6 years lost searching for solutions she kind of already knew. Could she have done it herself? Yes, probably, eventually, but her insights would have been harder to distinguish. Having me there making her curious by asking her powerful questions that she admitted were a total surprise, led her to the path of insight and realisation. This was her investment in me, which paid off big time, as it liberated her from despair and uncertainty. She did that when she got out of her own way.

She went looking for the wrong remedy, as so many people do. We are educated to only deal with symptomatic relief, and very rarely have the patience to understand the real cause. For sustainability and return of investment, this is the only way. My programme starts with coaching new awareness first, and if later down the line, we need a nutritionist or a personal training, I can give a whole solution and package that are add-ons, if they are relevant and needed at all.

The remedy Alice needed was someone to hold space for her, so that she could explore herself in depth in her own time—and naturally, that's very important—and work on her whole self, not just bits from this person and then another professional to work on that bit. It's so disjointed—how can that possibly work—she was not a business that needed fixing in this area or that area. She was like any one of us: a living, breathing, functionally complex and unique individual being. She told me that in those six years of searching for answers, she had four different practitioners working with her on various issues, and because they were so different, no advice or guidance was in synergy with the other, and all she did was go round and round. These issues did not budge until she was allowed to create a structure on living that made sense to her! Why? Because she created it herself, for herself, and the first point was for her to make a decision on going back to basics with her life, which was unnecessarily overcomplicated and needed drastic simplification. She could not interrupt the complex patterns of her life until she saw her own view from above—way above, like hovering in a helicopter—and until she saw herself and all the bits and pieces of her life that she had created in such a dysfunctional way. From there, she could see which parts she needed to deal with, one piece at a time, and not run from it. From here, she was her own master—the captain of her ship.

So let's go back to basics again. That is the initial platform for a long, healthy life, for you and your loved ones.

Question for you:
"What if you simplified parts of your life and your health?"

Guiding principle:
"If your foundation for living is contaminated and outdated,
it will pose a threat to you; break it down and start rebuilding
with better materials, aligned to your whole health."

The Good Old Days

My children run away when I start on this "back in my days" talk or discussion. I hope you don't run away, because there is some great value in comparative and insightful understanding of the good old days. Like I said before, I feel so lucky to have experience in both landscapes, and I am not even considered old! The wisdom from the past, my experiences, and that of all my clients put together, puts me in such an honoured and grateful position. I feel it is an important and serious duty to share this wisdom.

Our way of living is too complex in the West. Unfortunately, I can also see the Eastern side of our world catching up, but there are still many countries and communities that have withheld their culture and way of living, and seek to still pass that down. I like things to stay as traditional as is possible and not get amended and eroded to fit into modern culture. I know of so many Hindu practices and spiritual teachings that my culture and I like to share, but yet protect it from being misused or practiced in ways that take away its purity, innocence, and wisdom. Visitors want or need to modify it because then they can offer something unique and interesting to their market, like a business. There are some things that have to be protected in order to keep giving the correct purpose and meaning, but people are greedy—thieves even—and act like vultures, taking from sacred teachings on a global scale. The worst thing is that they don't give anything back to the country or people that shared it, and many in India, who have the wisdom, share through innocence, not knowing how or where this material is to be used. Some also give away wisdom for such a small price because they themselves also don't understand the real value of it. India, amongst so many other countries, are able to share of course, but they need to do it responsibly wherever they can, vetting people and organisations. For those who are drawn in to spend their money under the false illusion of something authentic, please validate it, vet it, and quality check it. If we were all just a bit more careful, things would automatically remain valuable and authentic, maintaining their rightful meaning, purpose, and authenticity. Let's back countries and people with great spiritual wisdom, history, and learned dimension—that kind of intellectual property has to be protected.

Today, our communities are broken and, in some cases, divided. We tend to mind our business a bit too much, and find it hard to ask and secure help when we really could use it. I acknowledge that these are generalisations, but our family framework is weaker because of it. Families are set up and encouraged to be independent, and because of that, the dynamics have changed, and not all for the better. There is much more pressure on women and men to do and be more, and because our parents and grandparents are living longer, we tend to be caretakers to them. They may also be living on their own, and we sometimes run three to four different households; whereas before, we all lived together and helped each other out. Now, I am not saying that we need to return to that. I think, for some of you, it would seem like a nightmare suggestion; but hopefully you understand that being together in a more meaningful way does have its benefits too.

I was born in Tanzania, East Africa, and I came into a big family, with grandparents, aunties, and uncles living with us. I was privileged to have hard-working parents and family members who lived in a beautiful house by the sea, and life was very much about outdoor living, social fun, and balanced living. The environment, as I remember very clearly, was inspiring and carefree, with so many stories and dreams shared with each other, being held emotionally, and supported and encouraged at every milestone I reached. But I was also encouraged to take part in charity and community events from a very young age. I was forever climbing trees and falling down, and talking to people that passed my home. It was a unique mix of freedom, not just because I was a child but because I saw the same thing in the way my parents and relatives lived. There was hardly any crime, and my parents were at home more than they were at work; in fact, my school started very early. I was in class at 7 a.m., and back home at 12 for lunch, with my parents and sister; and then sometimes I would go back to school after a quick nap, for crafts, sports, and vocational skills like cooking or woodwork, depending on a rotating timetable.

My parents also returned to work, and then they would be back home for 4 p.m., after which we would have a snack with tea and then all go to the beach together to meet friends and get some evening exercise. I was in bed by 7:30 p.m., and we would not eat a great deal in the evening; our main meal was lunch. How different our days are in the UK. We work from 8 a.m. in the morning till 6 p.m. at night, with interrupted lunch breaks, working lunches, and sometimes none at all; and then when home, it's too dark to do anything outside. We all eat a massive meal and sit in front of the television, and even if we do go out again, it's to a meal out or the cinema. But most are too tired to do this through the week, so it is reserved for weekends, which goes so quick because families have to cram so much in—homework, cleaning, some entertainment and socialising, shopping, and even weekend work tasks that had not gotten finished through the week. It is like a hamster living in a cage, going round and round on its hamster wheel.

I remember how important our family meals were, full of freshly cooked, healthy, wholesome foods, with no distractions apart from eating and meaningful talk and laughter about our morning and what plans we had for the afternoon. There was no hierarchy or head of the table that had control over the rest of us, but as a child, I had respect for my parents and grandparents. Everyone just got together like it was always meant to be, and I remember that we could rotate seats every day and sit where we liked. At the table, we were equal, and I had just as much to offer to adult conversations—they were mostly questions, as I tried to understand the big words and complex sentences, of course! We ate good, freshly prepared food in a relaxed fashion, with no clocks ticking or phones going off. We all then had a snooze to aid digestion and to be out of the sun for a while before returning to work or afternoon school. For extracurricular activities, like sports and craft workshops, I remember that I could choose, every 2 months, what I wanted to do. I was free enough to choose my own timetable to support my interests. The morning was spent doing the main academic subjects.

We would all return home by 4:30 p.m., and after some light refreshments, we would all jump in the car for time at the beach. Here we would talk, walk, meet friends, and generally be together, and if we felt like it, occasionally, we would get some street food, which was delicious as we rarely had too much to eat at night time, our main meal being lunch. Street food at the beach would include delightful fruit like mango with chili, charcoaled cassava, and so on. It was and still is, in my opinion, an idyllic life, and our unity with family and friends was incredible. I came to the UK at the age of ten, to pursue my natural interest in health, and what I thought in those days was only through a medical career. Here in the UK, in contrast to my earlier experiences of life in Africa, at just ten years of age, I experienced racism and bullying, long hours at school, and nothing to do outdoors after school. It was important to me to be in the UK for my studies and education. At the time, I was living with my aunty, who looked after me. My days on a beach were replaced with watching television or just doing homework. Kids need to be outside exploring, imagining, and dreaming—not cooped up near the television or tablet, eating junk mindlessly.

All the food I ate in Africa, I knew where it came from—its source, local trees and plants, vegetation, the fresh fish and seafood, as well as our meat, which were not factory farmed but grazed on grass and nearby pastures. How many children today in the West even know what they are eating or where it comes from, let alone how to even cook some basic things?

That lack of knowledge is such a disservice to them.

The good old days promoted more talking and connecting with each other, and telling stories to each other. I think it is so inspirational for an elder in the family to be teaching the younger ones something so important through storytelling. Humans have had this ritual of sitting all around the campfire, telling stories of before our modern world. That's how wisdom gets passed on. We don't have time for this now, not on a consistent basis, and even if we do, people rarely listen attentively. Why should they? There is always the internet for information, and so many people have so much ego that they can't surrender to themselves—they just don't know yet and need to learn. They think going to school or college just about covers it all. Social interaction from our elders must be preserved and encouraged. They are such a gift, but loneliness and the perception that they are a nuisance, makes them ill, fearful, and lonely.

That wisdom, if not passed on, will die with them. We don't have campfires that we gather round, but we do have a dinner table or somewhere to gather. That's where to do this and connect in a deeper way to each other.

The saying "quality time," which most parents know, me included, describes a special carved out time that you need to spend with each other. Some parents know that they don't spend any time with their children, so this "quality time" is misused and misguided—it is one more thing to add on to their to-do list; and like most to-do lists, things get put off. Having a family is more about *being*, not doing. They are all included and very much a part of your *being*, so spend time with people in a way that you can focus your whole attention on them, or include them in important areas of your life, without any distraction. It's a challenge I know, and yet vital. Is that not better than actually getting to the stage in your life where you have to diarise spending time with your loved ones. I involve my children in all decisions—and yes, that can be a headache—but I get their attention and their involvement from the beginning, and it is important for them to realise that the outcome evolves into something that may not be what they first thought of. That builds resilience and strength, and a way to acknowledge that they can be happy, because it is about working as a team on important issues that impact everyone, and we can all get pleasure from this.

The good old days promoted and encouraged cooking and using naturally grown raw ingredients to make home-cooked meals, and then spending time eating together at the dinner table. It was done mindfully when we valued tasting our food and having sufficient amounts to satisfy our physical hunger. It called for and allowed good eating habits, and it was also an opportunity to pass on and learn things from and about each other. It was an opportunity for communicating and spending social aspects of our lives together, even when it was done intuitively in complete silence because people were enjoying their food so much that they didn't really speak. And that wasn't a bad thing—in fact, it was healthy. Part of the problem today is that our eating has become so distracted that we don't feel satisfied with the food or the gesture of a family eating together, so we tend to overeat and miss the cues of satiety.

There is an obsession about eating until your belly is so full that it's painful. Just witness and observe people who go to all-you-can-eat buffets, where they pay a small price to get a ticket to overeat and pile their plates so high and wide that I wonder how they fit it all. It's the shiny deals and false perception of value for money, when you can eat as much as you want, and people get hooked on all that, and all rational grounded sense is left outside the door. It's the abundant feasting motivation, actually rooted in lack, which some call greed, but perhaps it's a bit of both. It certainly brings up the emotions as a consequence of thinking that "I am missing out." During the cavemen days, this was fine, because that one feast would last us for many days, without other possible sources of food, and that would allow the body to balance its energy stores. Today, we feast almost every day, and we don't allow our bodies time to use it up, so we store it instead, making us gradually fatter and sicker. Some of us can literally override the pain from overeating and a distended stomach, all for getting their money's worth in eating.

When we speak to each other, let's do it carefully and with love. Sometimes silence is a great way of communicating because it lets you just be. During the early era of black and white movies, there was no speech—just movement and expressive body language—but we still managed to work out the storyline and feel the emotions. Today, our world is filled with words—too many words, and unnecessary noise. We live overstimulated and out of balance.

We live in sad times, where it takes celebrity TV chefs to encourage good food in schools, only to find that most kitchen staff don't cook for themselves, and don't know anything about food and nutrition for the job.

The good old days also meant that we were so much more active. I may have had the attributes of a Hoover doing some cleaning for me, but I still had to do the dishes and scrub the floors, and there was a time when no gadgets were available to get the house, car, and garden tidy, apart from your own muscles doing the work. My father cleaned his cars and never used the cleaning stations. There was movement and activity. Doing something meant that we had to physically move our bodies. The convenience age now means that we have every gadget and gizmo available to do the work for us, rendering our minds and bodies—which are purposely designed, biological machinery— into redundancy.

Another observation from the good old days is that we were not encouraged to take every medicine available for anything. Nowadays, we do not trust our bodies enough, and don't let them do what is needed to counteract any illness. We rush to the pharmacist or to the doctor, pushing for pills and potions so that we don't have to spend too much time being ill or feeling ill. Whereas I like that motivation, I think it's not entirely genuine if we are to return to the type of lifestyle that doesn't keep us sick and therefore needing more medicine; we have some work to do. Leave the vicious circle and find a way out.

It is normal, every now and again, to catch a cold, or have pain somewhere; it is a way that your body signals to you to take note and respond, to correct your life balance. But people actually abuse this signaling by taking unnecessary medicine that just makes their bodies lazy. No one is invincible, and any illness can be a shock. Let me tell you that using fast track measures to fix this is also an illusion, and in many cases, you will be barking up the wrong tree. Prescription antibiotics is one group of medicine that has been over-prescribed, and they are not having the same effect as they did before, because organisms like bacteria and viruses can develop and change to respond to them. Antibiotics have a detrimental effect on our gut microbiome, which is one key area to protect when it comes to appropriate defenses, immunity, and other important physiological functions like hormone regulation and inflammatory markers. This is largely the problem with current lifestyle diseases like gut issues, diabetes, and cardiovascular components.

Our doctors were different in the service they gave us when I was young. Now it takes a few weeks before you can even get an appointment to see your GP here in the UK. Waiting times for surgery are high, and the general demand for our healthcare service is so high that it is not coping and radically needs updating. Part of family wisdom is no longer shared, or if shared, not valued as tried and tested, because we are so sold on the fact that doctors know it all—or we trust Google.

The list of ingredients that I was taught to cook with, like turmeric, cumin, ginger, garlic, and many more amongst the list of herbs and spices, made our food really tasty but also packed nature's health in every spoonful, and what is completely natural to me now seems to be a marketable commodity amongst others who are searching for its benefits in a more commercial way. Whilst I encourage the harnessing of such wisdom and the enterprise shown, it is missing key pieces because it's the combination of ingredients that make up the optimal benefit, and knowing how to use them to get food tasty and delicious, whilst keeping it healthy, is an ancient skill. The food that you get in eateries is not what I am talking about. This food I talk about is homemade from fresh and basic ingredients, and I am proud to be a part of this wisdom; but it is dying, and I want to preserve this knowledge of food as the medicine for today and tomorrow.

There is so much value in the good old days, and just like fashion, it comes round again. I think this is our time to reconnect to it in a new way.

Question for you:
"What can you remember from the good old days that can be part of your life today? Ask the elders for their perspectives."

Guiding principle:
"It is elements of the good old days—when our food was healthy,
our soil was rich in nutrients that grew our fruit and vegetables,
and we made time to cook—that will bring us out of this
ill health void we are in today."

Early Intervention

When it comes to health and wellbeing, we tend to be reactive rather than proactive. I know we tend to encourage exercise and eating well, but that's really all we do; and honestly, if we did not get information on why it is important and how to do it, from government or public health institutions, we probably would not have it on our minds. Our dimension for health and wellbeing has primarily been on fitness, exercise, and diet. Thank goodness we have started to understand that it is not enough. Actually, all these aspects, and more that are covered here in this book, have to be connected to give a cumulative result of sustainable wellbeing. I hope this gives you a more potent and lasting impression for my desire for you, for a true and complete health and wellbeing blueprint. More need for better mental health is being recognised because of the obvious increase in mental health and stress-related issues, and we also know that so many are sick today despite knowledge and intervention and facilities, so there are pieces to the puzzle that are obviously missing and not being dealt with. That's where I come in. You cannot have or strive for balance without knowing the true story.

For the typical average family with a modest income and two children, it is a challenge these days to pay attention to health in a way that is easy and lasting, which also, by the way, goes way beyond the focus for sugar-free foods, although that is helpful but not the entire picture. We know that families are bigger in numbers now, through the increase in second or third marriages. Roles are being created in family settings where each person knows their perspective focus and influence on the family (e.g., breadwinner, cook, head of the family, etc.) As the saying goes, too much of anything is no good and results in an imbalance in something else. So we need to nurture a proactive and wholesome approach to health in our lives and be less reactive, as a real and lasting solution for our present and future health.

We gain our influential thoughts from external sources in the first place. These influences are from people inside and outside our homes, the media, government incentives, and the health and wellness industry that we cannot tune into for what we know and trust. There is so much noise in this industry, and I hope that this book sets a precedent that health is personal and goes far beyond being fit and eating healthy. I want you to work on what you need, and work on the different layers contained in this book. There are no false claims here; much of it is my truth and the truth of all my clients. It is important to me that you take full responsibility for your health and get to know yourself and what your body and mind are capable of.

We work much harder than before in supporting our careers, families and social commitments, so we don't always have the time and space to requalify our health and wellbeing. Let's put it at the heart of our life strategy, because it will serve you in ways not ever imagined. It is, as you are finding out, the most crucial building block, and it needs to be called forth much earlier on in our lives. I want that to be at the beginning of life—parents-to-be and each and every one of us needs to lead by example. It won't be perfect, but as long as it is a conscious effort, that is enough. Great health has a leadership quality and can inspire and support you in whatever you experience in life. You can lean into it, and it will hold you every step of the way. Good health has your back always.

I know the challenge of keeping an eye on health with so many other aspects of life needing our attention, but this is not about perfection here; instead, it's about knowing balance and an imbalance, and jumping in quickly to resolve the latter before it becomes a problem. If you don't pay it timely attention, then it will hinder you in more ways than you could ever know, and show up at the most inconvenient points in time. Imagine all the good things that can happen, like setting off to travel the world, or entering into a major deal at work, getting married and having children, and so on—true life pleasures—only for it to be spoilt by the inconvenience of failing health, like an ache that once was a quiet signal to you, which got ignored and has just got louder, and has now stopped you in your tracks. It does not have to be that way. You would not ignore squeaky brakes for your car, would you? Our bodies are also mechanistic, and the unique engineering that goes into our working body is vital for being alive; yet we ignore it, because we can—for now anyway. Are we less important than our cars?

In reality, you know what happens. Appointments with health practitioners get delayed or cancelled by you, and you manage to get by with painkillers. You continue your daily routine without the reminders to stop and be mindful. Pain continues, and you continue to ignore it, with the help of codeine. Why is that? Our choice is wealth over health; after all, it's not urgent enough. When urgent becomes acute, that's the risk you take daily—a silent and yet patient ticking bomb. No one knows you are suffering; it may show weakness, so it is better to carry on! Our expectation of health in us and others is so low. Why do we tolerate aches and pains, headaches, and digestive issues every day? It's a sign for you that something somewhere in your body is not at its best. We have been taught to ignore it because it's a sign of weakness and vulnerability; instead, what happens is that we brave up and get on, which is trained into us as strength. What absolute rubbish. There is nothing stronger than love, for yourself and others. That's intelligence, so stop and pay attention, and seek help and guidance within yourself. It will give you true insight of what is happening in the moment, and that's all we have: the now, the present, without which we cannot tell the difference between our past and future.

Health is our wealth, not the other way around, but YOU can HAVE BOTH.

In reality, we will get sick every now and again, but that's not the same as radical changes that give rise to disease—chronic disease that is there to take hold. We all catch colds or catch things when we come across a new environment or people, and that's okay; our bodies are equipped well to cope with any minor acute illness. The test is not so much that you are ill, but the ability to recover quickly using only your inherent systems without the use of conventional medicine. I believe and have proved that chronic disease can be reversed, and balance and harmony brought back into your body's physiology and workings. We are just all too quick to remedy things with all sorts of pain killers and counter remedies rather than allowing the time for our bodies to recover themselves, or doing what we can intellectually to address its need without running to the health practitioner. In the long term, it makes us reliant and actually weakens us. I like the idea of restorative health.

If you are having a heart attack or stroke, call 999 emergency line. That's appropriate, and it's the urgency of such things that is the dance between living and dying. That's not what I am talking about. I know you know that, but I thought it best to just point that out before we go on.

Early intervention is something I am very passionate about, so it becomes part of family values in every culture, like food is an integral part of all our lives but is not the full story. We need to eat to live, not live to eat, as the saying goes. There are functional reasons for good wholesome nutritious food that is a physiological need for each of us, but because of TV and media, advertisement, the food industry cutting corners or getting in on market trends set by the dieting industry, or even public health (like "low fat," "low or zero sugar"), we have become obsessed with food, and the part it plays in our lives is way bigger than it needs to be.

We have been talking about food, good and bad, healthy and unhealthy, and fat and sugar and this and that, for too long—I am frankly so bored of it—we need to move on, really. I don't think doing nutrition courses are worthy, because they follow the guidelines set by institutions anyway, and if the guidelines are not updated, they are misleading. Like everything that is a trend, it comes and goes, and nutrition today is a big trend—tomorrow, it will be something else. I want to give health a bigger view that is not trend related or controlled by a few influential people in health, but the key to unlocking your own unique health. We need to move on and simplify food, which is about getting people back in touch with sourcing food, and educating people on foods—where it comes from; having community farms, where each of us can grow our own fruits and vegetables, and share the crops so that food is picked and eaten quickly from its natural habitat, rather than it sitting in fridges wrapped in plastic. We need to learn to cook the basic staples again, and also healthy, stunning food for entertainment and the social aspect.

We need to learn to quickly recognise ingredients and foods when we are eating out. We need to learn to manage portions and not get greedy, just because we can. To me, cake is cake, and I expect it to have butter and sugar when I eat it, but I can choose to moderate my eating of cake. I don't want to pick up cake laced with crap and artificial sweeteners and additives just because it says the calories are low. I know that when I eat cake every now and again, there is no harm, so please people, come off this silly calorie-controlled movement. Eat real food. Cook real food. Share real food. I don't buy cake that has sat on shelves. I make it myself; it is the simplest thing, and I know what ingredients go into it. My cakes have sugar, butter, and flour and eggs—that's it, four ingredients—there is no real harm from those ingredients as it is apportioned to one slice, but keep an eye on it.

But we are made to feel guilty, so we eat more. Guilt is a waste of time and can cause more harm in our eating patterns than eating in moderation and mindfully, and if you cannot do it on your own, then get help. Compare a homemade cake with one bought in and already made commercially. There will be more than the necessary four ingredients of a basic cake, because it needs to sit on the shelf for a long time before it is picked and consumed. By then, it is usually tasteless and dry. This calorie restriction by conventional dieting methods is beyond boring and is, at best, the biggest disillusionment of our time. It creates a very awkward and unhealthy relationship with food. We do not want to be passing this way on to our kids. Instead, we need to teach them very simply and clearly about boundaries with moderation, educating them and teaching them to makes simple, quality, wholesome meals that are both cost effective and tasty. Today, new mums don't always have the skills and the patience to cook for themselves. It is always more attractive to buy in to such time-poor individuals and those that have higher disposable income. By the time they have thought of what to buy, gone to the shops, picked up a dozen extra things not on the list, I would have cooked three wholesome meals for my family.

Here is the thing; there is always time, but how we choose to use it tells us apart.

The harm comes from the daily assault of sugary foods that people eat and crave. My concern with the movement against sugar is the same that happened with fats, and look where that got us: in a worse position. It's more important to understand and educate on choosing foods that don't contain sugar, rather than replacing sugar with sugar alternatives and calling them healthy when they are not—counting calories and skipping nutrition is never healthy. So don't go there! Stick to whole foods; there is automatic portion control that way too. Two whole dates are better than a dose of date syrup! We all need to be conscious of glycaemic load, whether we are diabetic or not. Your liver and pancreas as are other organs are meant to serve you your entire life. Don't abuse them just because you have no illness that shows up at this moment.

Let's not make this mistake. Let's instead bake cakes and biscuits at home if we really have to. Let's get back to seeing fruits, vegetables, and butchers, instead of gigantic supermarkets where we are enticed to buy far more than we need, and to fall foul to the tricks of the marketeers.

If you or your children need to stop eating too much sugar, then learn to deal with its addiction and make better choices instead. Do not think that sugary foods are treats. How many times in your life have you perceived something sweet as a reward or a treat? That's what you need to deal with—it's the psychology that needs correcting.

This intervention starts early when you start being weaned off milk as a baby. Taking the culprit food away is not a way forward, because you crave it even more, but having a healthy relationship with sugar is best, and there is a proven way of doing this. It is better to stick to the real deal than to replace it with alternatives. Good psychology with food is key, and a healthy relationship with food only starts early. The biggest lesson is not to make a fuss with our little ones, or they will rebel when they are teenagers, and you will wonder what the hell you did wrong. I have cooked healthy, wholesome food every day for my children, apart from when we were on holiday, and then it is about management and choosing healthier lists off the menu, not justifying having a break from healthy eating just because you are on holiday. That is called the binge culture, which so many are afflicted with today—with food, with drink, and with anything that can become addictive in time. You will not miss out on anything when you live in a balanced way, but if you treat food in treat and non-treat forms, then you will, and that's what the dieting industry has done—it makes us feel guilty.

Our perception of what is good and bad food needs to change, especially when many food companies and many of the biggest dieting programme brands have products that have heavily processed ingredients in the products. Yes, they are low in calories, but the real cost of substituting calories with artificial ingredients is madness. Why? Yet they win tender after tender from local councils in order to spread their myths and hook more people in the name of community weight loss.

We question each other on whether we have eaten or not, so why not question how much "me" time was given to yourself today, or what exercise you did today. It is about creating the right environment in our families, paying attention mindfully to every moment in our lives, creating a strategy and testing it, and changing it or maintaining it wherever and whenever needed. Now, I am not one to promote "one size fits all." What I talk about here is much deeper: It's making health and wellbeing part of our fabric of life. Being consistent with it, leading by example, and including everyone in the household is so important, so that it becomes what they expect and are part of. When younger, they learn how to include it so that they don't struggle to choose it whilst other aspects of their lives evolve. It is about teaching it to our young people, because simply doing it yourself does not always guarantee that others will follow in your pursuit. Instead, it is about each of us being responsible for our own health and wellbeing, and making each other accountable for their own, and then also adding a level of fun, adventure, and laughter to it, such as bike rides, eating and cooking together, talking about shopping together, choosing food together and opening up conversation on its benefits, and letting them choose what is right for them, from a good source of healthy pursuits and interests.

Early intervention has to be empowering rather than dictatorial nagging noise. I have known families who were always telling their children to run around outside and play, and go do this or that, whilst all they did was sit around and never exercised themselves; or when they did, it was accompanied by disempowering statements like, "I hate by body," "It is hard work," "Skinny people are lucky; they eat and drink what they like," "I was not made for exercise," and "I hate vegetables." The list of such statements is endless. What are yours that automatically get verbalised when triggered in a certain way or setting? Are they empowering to you and others, or not? Are they even true when you think about them very carefully?! Or is it mindless banter that needs to stop?!

We do really need to very carefully choose what we say around anyone who is influenced by us, but we complicate this when it is actually quite simple. In the example above, these children may do it for you in the short run, but as soon as they can stop, they will. This way of communication is not empowering but reactive and disempowering, and is unsustainable through the course of that child's life, and that is what we don't want. No matter what life's journey we experience, health and wellbeing will be our very foundation from which everything else is built and maintained.

This will reap rewards if you can encourage them to empower themselves and look after themselves in all areas of health and wellbeing. We have all met that one person who is so empowered in their health that firstly it is second nature, and thoughts like, "I will do it tomorrow," or, "It's raining; I can't go for a run," does not even enter their minds. It is more like they acknowledge that running in the rain is not their preference, but if they were to look at the forecast, they could negotiate when they could go. They make the effort to adhere the best they can with their goals, and manage their internal dialogue well enough so that it does not get sabotaged through justified reasoning. They are motivated, and more importantly, clearly understand the reasons, benefits, and purpose to their ways. It is with ease that they live this way—relaxed and not uptight—just as automatic and effortless as brushing their teeth in the morning.

I have had some fun with some workshops I did in temples here in the UK. Temples are a centre for worship, as well as community centres, where education is important on various aspects of life. This particular event was for singles looking to match themselves to someone for marriage and unity. These young adults and their parents acknowledge that it is not as easy to complement each other, and it is hard to find a suitable match, more so today than ever, and singles are becoming fussy in what they want. What most people are on the lookout for are looks, the initial attraction, financial position, professional work and ability for future or current wealth, and dedication to religion. What is still missing is how they look after themselves, because being youthful doesn't stay like that forever. What goals would they have for children in the manner of health? It does not come up in conversation. We think that if we look okay on the outside, then our health must be okay. Not necessarily! Girls in particular need to be taught this, especially after marriage, because in most cases, they have been groomed to look their best for their match. Unfortunately, it is a tick in the box exercise, and a superficial one at that. Without health and wellbeing in that person, and for both in unity of marriage, this will not be a priority to their children; it will still be the typical default attributes of profession, wealth, religion, and status that will get passed down to measure against. I know this to be true in many cases, and that's a part of my culture that is not ideal and needs to change. Chasing all that will actually compromise their health eventually. It does, and still they do the same things again and again.

I recently heard of a singles matching agency that matched people using fitness. I thought this was a great idea!

Question for you:
"If you could claw back time to your younger years,
what intervention in health would you put into place
that would be really valuable to you today?"

Guiding principle:
"Teach health, talk health, and be health from start to finish."

Healthy Boundaries

Living by boundaries is what we mostly do, if you think about it. Some of them are not ones you have chosen but are present to help with your living experience. It gives you a little guidance. There are laws of the land, driving rules and working ethics and regulations, just as some examples of some boundaries. Each of us will have some important boundaries that govern the way we live and what is important to us. Some of us have not heard of making boundaries in our personal lives, yet we do this for our work lives, especially boundaries that are thought through, chosen with the aim to be effective. I do know, however, people who live their lives through very rigid boundaries, and lack spontaneity, which have made them slaves, and it can feel like a miserable existence if not careful and regularly updated.

By now, you will know that I am a fan of something in the middle—that notion called balance. I tend to move away from dissonance and seek to live by what is important and healthy for myself, and also for the people that mean so much to me and are affected by my choices. I cannot encourage myself in ways that I don't encourage in others.

Healthy boundaries in aspects of our lives help us to organise and compartmentalise things for our benefit. When you choose boundaries that are healthy to you, then you can feel safe and supported and actually guided by it. The important preliminary to setting boundaries is to think it through, and to understand its benefits to you and how it can shape your life because of the benefits. There are some areas where boundaries need to be flexible, or rigid yet timely.

We all know the "diets don't work" tune. It may enlighten you to know that they do work, but it's the boundaries that you have around the diet that brings results, or in most cases, no significant results. For someone who plays that tune of, "Oh, this diet did not work for me," ask them why. Most come up with a barrage of excuses: "It made me miserable," or "I could not stick to it." The power to assert yourself has always been with you, not the diet. It's like they choose to do the diet and then they go and make up their own rules but still expect the results from the original set-up, and when they know they cannot get away with it, and the results are affected, they get a bout of remorse because of their actions, and then blame it on the diet or blame something or someone else.

The problem is that most diets only deal with the nutritional or fitness angle, and not many deal with the self-development and awareness angle, which is the start of where you really understand what and who you are, and how you may be challenged in this diet if at all. Most people just fall into dieting mode without really thinking about the consequences—positively or negatively—and so are not ready or prepared for what it may bring. Here is a typical example for a dieting candidate that has a good few pounds to lose at the start of the new year, along with many others with such resolutions to get leaner and fitter, or for a holiday six months away. Well, it starts with excitement and a good deal of motivation, cutting this and that out to get that slimmer body, and exercising a little more to keep the momentum up and get you nearer the expected results. Then for some reason, you hit a hard week at work, and your need to pop open a bottle of wine to relax is higher on the agenda at that time, so you relax the restriction a little for a day. But then you notice that you need that to get past the whole weekend, and then, on Monday, you just can't get back to that place of your intentions for a slimmer body. Then a friend invites you out for a catch-up social, involving food and drinks, and you go and partake fully. However, what becomes apparent when you reflect over the past few weeks is that you have had too many time-out sessions from your regime, and your motivation to stick to losing that weight starts to become a little diluted and much harder.

A few weeks in, usually the middle of January, after having those little cheats and cutting corners, suddenly the results you wanted (i.e. losing some weight) have flat lined, and it's becoming harder. And you are yet again on the brink of giving in, because the results are not matching the amount of effort and fight that is going into getting back to the clean eating or whatever else you are on—it's not worth continuing because it does not work! You can hear the dialogue in your head that justifies why you couldn't do it—right?

However, if you had kept to your boundaries that were in alignment to your goal in this area, then it would have worked. In my experience, most dieters do it alone, which gives rise to many problems on their journey because they are not aware of anything about themselves at all. There are many practitioners who deliver their own dieting programmes but have never been fat themselves. They have good intentions, I am sure, but they lack the insight and foresight for their clients, as they have no experience of it and simply cannot understand what they are going through. They try to relate, but without the necessary experience of that, they really just can't, and they become just as desperate to fix this as their clients.

If you decide that you want a clean month, then specify exactly what "clean" means—for example, no alcohol, no sugar. Whatever it is that you know you need to do to get a result, then do it and stick to it. When a party invite with alcohol and cakes pops up, go by all means, but you don't have to eat or drink inappropriately just because it's an invitation and people feel sorry for you. In my years of experience, I have met many ignorant people who feel sorry for people who decide they want to do something for better health. They can sabotage you, be very critical of what you are trying to achieve, and absolutely stand in your way with their one dimensional and ignorant opinion. To encourage someone—truly encourage someone—they need to get over themselves.

Such circumstances will test your commitment, and it is only when accepting your commitment through boundaries, that you will be serious. Think of all areas of your life where you have boundaries (a line or fencing around), and all sorts of examples in other areas of your life where you set boundaries that work well for you, and ones that are incorrectly set or are non-existent. Every successful area of each person will have appropriate boundaries to help them stay focused and steer them away from temptations or even people that have different boundaries, which may impact on yours in a negative way. Losing weight comes from well-chosen boundaries and internal motivation; without one or the other, it's futile. And here is the thing: Forget about starting any weight loss programme in January; it's futile and riddled with hardship and sabotage. I turn people away in January, and I start in February—I can then combine two months into one, with motivation and results.

Think of our best athletes and what boundaries they have in place, through their daily living, that gets them their ultimate triumph: a gold medal for being the best and fastest in the world, and in the headlines.

Sticking to your boundaries also has a phenomenal impact on the relationship you have with yourself. You begin to trust yourself and believe in what you can achieve. I mean, how powerful is that?

Can you think of times when you have broken boundaries and what chain of events has followed, including the way you thought or felt afterwards for a day or two?

Be specific in setting boundaries, so that they have clarity. I have been asked if they are like goals, and my answer is that if you have a goal, then think of that, the outcome you want, and then set yourself boundaries in terms of what you need to do to achieve it. Boundaries you set must serve you, even though initially it may be uncomfortable to stick to the framework; but with time and through seeing some good results, your faith in them begins to increase, and it becomes non- negotiable to break or bend them until you are ready. And even then, that may just be to tweak them to carry you further along.

Remember that they can be adjusted when necessary, as long as the adjustment is taking you forward and is not used as an excuse to sabotage you in any way. They cannot be ridiculous and hard to live by, causing you to rebel against these boundaries. Setting boundaries that are too rigid may not be appropriate for the goal, so align your boundaries to the aim; they can be rigid if that is what it will take, or flexible to a degree.

See the difference between rules and boundaries, according to the definitions:

Rules –

- One set of explicit or understood regulations or principles governing conduct or procedure within a particular area of activity.
- Control of or dominion over an area or people.
- Exercise ultimate power or authority over (an area and its people).
- Pronounce authoritatively and legally to be the case.

Boundaries –

- A line that marks the limits of an area; a dividing line.
- A limit of something abstract, especially a subject or sphere of activity.

A business man Tony, who was desperate to get fitter and healthier decided to join a gym in his local area, and he decided to use this as his "me" time every day for an hour so. It was his goal to get fitter by getting to the gym seven days a week for an hour. There is no debating the clarity of this mission, although there could be a little more clarity and specifics as to what fitter and healthier looks like for him, so that he could at least recognise it when it comes about. However, what he discounted at the very first hurdle was that his work diary was very busy. It was too busy, and he was regularly being called away to work, which was the problem in the first place, and the reason for his diminishing health. His activities took him away, travelling on other people's timelines. His work was so important to him, and he enjoyed it, so he never felt that it was wrong to devote so much of himself to it. Like so many of us, I am sure we can relate. What would he have needed to do with asserting his boundaries, in order to get to the gym seven days a week? Do you think he succeeded?

Yes, he needed to free up an hour a day for himself, which he felt was doable and also necessary to claim some work-life balance. He knew that even when travelling, all his hotels had gyms, so there was no excuse. What he chose to do was to use his time to go to the gym for that hour, but bearing in mind that he wasn't going to the gym at all, he may have rushed his decision to claim back an hour and then also get himself to the gym at the same time for all of seven days. Was that realistic or a fantasy? As he experienced the challenge, he found it difficult to uphold the boundaries of giving himself one hour each day for seven days, never mind getting himself somewhere else too. He experienced others in his work schedule demanding his time, and he found it difficult to say no to them. Is that not the same challenge that so many of us face today? And because of this, he only managed to go once a week, which by the way is amazing considering he was not going at all. So even if he did not win against the challenge of seven times per week, what he did do is realise and become aware that he also had a responsibility to himself, not just his work colleagues, to keep his word for himself. He thought of another plan and encountered a simpler regime that allowed him to create a lifestyle that was inclusive of the things that were important to him, and also found that he was flexible enough about giving himself "me" time whilst abroad, where getting to the gym despite it being a few floors down in the same building was less motivating.

What Tony held on to was that one hour per day was for himself, where he could do what he wanted for himself, and that had a varied range of getting fitter and healthier. He went for walks at lunch time, or a stroll in the park before he went home, so you can see that he was holding his boundaries but also had the flexibility of how he chose and carved out time, depending on where he was and what he felt like doing. He also did get to the gym regularly but noticed after a while that there was more pleasure in walking in the park or at lunch times. We are not meant to be slaves to boundaries; they can be flexible. It's deciding on what is non-negotiable first, and what can have some degree of flexibility. Boundaries are there to keep things simple and structured, but they need to serve you appropriately and healthily.

Question for you:
"What boundaries do you have that serve your best health and what needs to be created?"

Guiding principle:
"Your boundaries that serve you are just that;
they are yours, and no one else has business there."

Lead by Example

Encouraging someone to get up, get fit, turn up to gym sessions or eat healthily, is a little more than just barking out orders and hoping that they do it.

In fact, the latter is the worst thing to do. Remember the earlier points, on rebellion? Remember the triggers that cause it in an unhelpful way? That's right; that's orders with criticism, critical and rigid rules, and mixed perception and messages! Rather, health and wellbeing have to be about choice and autonomy, not rules. The best way to encourage others in their health and wellness is to do it for yourself first, so that they see you walking the walk, and they see a benefit. I have seen firsthand too many parents that bark out orders to their children about eating healthily, and about exercising and getting out of the house, when they themselves were not complying with that lifestyle in any significant way. Instead, many children are told not to eat crisps, when they have caught their parents doing exactly that. Many eat those things in secret for fear of being found out.

No, I am not joking; secret eating is a very real issue for many—and not just away from the children but also partners, the public, and even work colleagues. It gives way to mixed messages. These can be disempowering, and lack respect and credibility. Many kids may follow the rule begrudgingly, but as soon as they don't have to follow this rule, they will break it, and with a huge feeling of ultimate freedom, which can be really unhelpful. What we surely want for them is to be rational and make decisions thoughtfully; so what we do with them when they are young, and how, is vitally important. Good, positive early years, being taught by leaders as an example, is what makes superb, grounded people.

When you lead by example, you show them and not just tell them. We model the behaviour, sets of actions, and way of lifestyle we want for each other. They need to see you doing the same things as what you tell them to do. In a family setting, there are too many rules that are for one and not for the other, and as much as I believe in accepting that to a degree and in some aspects of life, it is not appropriate for health and wellbeing. It has to be consistent for it to work out well.

I was not raised that way. Yes, I had boundaries for my safety and comfort, but I was included in all the main decisions and situations that unfolded in my parents' lives, which also affected me, and I had a say even at 3 years old! I was valued even when I was a kid. Health and wellness is one major area in our lives that we need to keep hold of at all times, so it's best done with collective congruency, authenticity, and consistency. These days, as you know, there are too many rules about what to eat and what not to eat, how to exercise, how to sleep, and what friends you need to keep and get rid of. Then there are rules from your boss; and kids have their teachers screaming and telling them to do this and that, giving detention for just going to the toilet during class—it's madness. We encourage madness in each other. In all this chaos, how can love ever show up the way it is meant to?

Lead by example, and lead with love for yourself and others; knowing what you want in your health and wellness will open you up to wanting the same for everyone else. I coached groups of women who struggled to show their vulnerability of eating unhealthily because they had to show and become a role model for their kids. It was a true eye opener, and so many noticed that their unhealthy bouts of eating had to go underground, get hidden, and be secretive, so that their husbands and partners and their kids would not see them doing it. They felt such shame, and this is just the kind of pressure that we cannot endure—it makes us sick!

I am against this because it's unnecessary, and there are better ways, where you can openly eat and drink mindfully, without shame.

There are certain aspects of your life where things are wonderful, and you will notice how that part in you was once led by example. If there is anyone in your friend or family circle that you admire for their health and wellbeing, ask them how they do it, and be led by their actions and habits. Start there and then, and when you do it for yourself, you will also get the opportunity to lead by example for your troop. If you don't, that is not a problem, because you can be your own example and lead from there. But just one thing: Choose people to share it with you that are willing to listen. We often choose the hardest of people and lose motivation when we can't change them, or they just cut us off, asking us to mind our business. Start easy and gain momentum first—the hardy, stubborn, self- important and sometimes ignorant ones will come round when they seek it. Sometimes they might not at all! That's okay.

If you are a parent reading this right now, or wanting to be, or you have some influence on children somewhere in your life, then we can do right by them. Raising healthy, happy, grounded children is not something that is automatic and easy; it's a highly skilled trait, and no one teaches us that in whole. Without attending courses and reading books on it, we simply learn by making mistakes, and regrettably, some don't learn from mistakes. Instead, they seek to blame others for the results and circumstances—that is their reason, always! Of course, as you would have read in the section about the good old days, this would have been passed on by the wise elders and families of our communities, whom we now don't engage with as much, and we live apart even though we may all live under one roof. I know that can have its barriers and problems to modern life being comfortable enough, especially when elders are stuck in their old, outdated and unhelpful ways, but pure wisdom is not about good or bad. You have to have the wisdom to see good in all scenarios.

Remember that if you have a hand in anything, and whatever the results, the outcome has your contribution.

People often wonder why our followers don't listen to us. It is because we live in a one-dimensional world, where what we could be doing is to be just blindly barking inconsistent orders at people we want to influence, without discussing the benefit. It is a reactive strategy. We can be reacting to our own displeasures or our own battles, and blindly passing them on. This is a classic example of the rise in obesity. It is a system of learning and teaching that gets passed on. The thoughts and behaviours are systemically passed on without even realising it. It's like a masterclass. The first step is to look at your learning and what and who you are, and then start there so that you are mindfully only passing on things that will be of service to others, because it comes through consciousness and not through being on autopilot mode.

To truly lead by example is to first learn about yourself through self-awareness, self-knowledge, and patterns of behaviours, and those all-important hidden beliefs that dictate your ways, so that you can check in with what you want to keep and what is so outdated and maybe doesn't even belong to you, which was transplanted as if by magic into the depths of your subconscious mind—like an invisible force.

A good example to demonstrate what I am saying is when I got our first family dog. It was actually a gift from a past client who knew I was thinking of getting a dog. Anyway, as a dog owner novice, I got to thinking about some obedience training for him, and I decided to take him to dog obedience classes. The trainer said to me, "The training is more about training YOU, not the dog. If you want a dog to behave in a way that is acceptable, then it will be YOU that will need training. He will not follow your lead without consistency; know what you want for him and yourself first."

He continued, "Most people can't hack the training because it feels like an assault on their ego. It's got nothing to do with the dog. They miss something about themselves; perhaps it's blind to them. It's mostly boundaries and consistency in the messages given to the dog."

I learnt and have known for some time that I cannot lead from my ego; it needs to be from my heart.

So what changes are you facilitating for yourself that will be felt in others as inspiring and impactful?

Alone, I cannot change the world to a better place of wellbeing—I need your help. Everyone needs to join in.

It's about giving every individual autonomy, to create the changes they want and that are right for them. As a leader, you don't want these people tied to you; they need to rise with you, and even overtake you, to be leaders in their own right.

Let me remind you of the purpose of this book: to hold on to health and wellness in a way that life events cannot break. Let's not fall for the voices that tell us that we don't have time, that there is too much going on, or that we need to fix this or that, before we can concentrate on ourselves. You cannot help anyone until you help yourself. Do that, and all is clear; don't do it, and you seek invisibility and dissonance.

We know it takes effort to renegotiate our commitments to it. As a mother, I know how hard it was and is to do anything for myself; whereas before, without them, it was so easy. I love my children, and the sacrifice, for a short time, was what it was. I have no regrets but joy that I held myself with patience and kindness and strength. The thing is not to fight it, but instead creatively think of how we can include what we want for them. Yes, it is a change, but whilst paying attention to the current situation and triggers you may be experiencing. Most of us tend to negotiate it completely for blocks of time in an all or nothing way. Then, of course, when I did have the time, I started to overthink, because that was my procrastinator strategy for not wanting to make an effort in my own health. I just got lazy! "I am too tired; I won't have time; I need to cook for the children; my kids are not well, and I can't leave them."

Lead by example so that you have the true and inspiring influence deserving for all.

Question for you:
"Think and write down all the mixed messages
about health and life that you give."

Guiding principle:
"Correct leadership is homegrown in a loving, compassionate
environment—that's your testing ground—be aware of your ways."

Consistency

It is the key to getting results you want and getting them quicker. I have to say that this is one I struggle with the most. I am a spontaneous character, and because of high intuitive prowess, consistency is placed toward the back of my toolkit. However, reflecting on all the things I have achieved, I have to admit that this may have started as an intuitive calling forth, but it was the practice of consistency, once I had committed, that got the idea to a physical manifestation, even though it took a few good years to get this book to this point, published, and in your hands.

Once the practice of consistency is attained, then results follow fast, and positive outcomes, benefits, and the feeling of happiness, achievement, and pride will surface, giving you the momentum to use the practice again in something else you want to achieve. The art and practice of consistency is both duplicable and sustainable.

For health and wellbeing to be sustainable and a part of everyday living, it will always be about consistent practice in some appropriate regard. One thing I have noticed in myself over the years, when I was not being consistent and therefore not getting the results I desired, was that the energy I spent in procrastinating or making excuses to not do something, was totally wasted. I noticed how much greater the energy was to not do something because my mind was involved in justifications and excuses, than the energy to just do it! Have you noticed something like that in yourself?

So, what is best for getting consistency in MOTION? It is momentum we are trying to achieve, heading in the direction of your choice. So, think about what you want to achieve in your health and wellbeing, and what you want as a result. Next, feel the emotion associated with its success and achievement, and then once you are able to see clearly what it is like to experience the benefits, then think of your strategy and what actions you need to take—just the first three crucial steps whilst holding on to the outcome you desire. What are you being? Are you being strong and persistent? Do you believe in yourself? Are you positive, energetic, and determined? Would that help you?

How?

Consistency in anything you want to achieve is crucial. It's like an easy flow toward your achievement. If your life is tainted with illness and disease, guess what? You have consistently done whatever to achieve this, and we are really good at consistently doing bad things and then wondering why that happened.

Sadly, our lives are full of inconsistencies, messages, behaviours, actions, and thoughts. Managing our mind is the thing to do in order to live well in today's world, and to keep it open enough to keep learning is the challenge. The deal with today's education is not progressive, as the curriculum is not balanced for life after school. All children need to be taught early how to master their mind. Then they will experience health and wellness for themselves, with ease and a peaceful flow. They really will!

So again, let me pose the question of what you want for your own health and wellness, and your life and that of others, which includes loved ones and the greater world. Where do we start this journey?

The next point is the starting point and a fundamental step to your journey. With this, you will go far in pursuit of your best health; without it, you will stay where you are, and as the world moves forward, you may even get left behind—always catching up but never leading and doing it with others. It's your choice.

I cover consistency in more detail later on.

Question for you:
"How are you with consistency?"

Guiding principle:
"Consistency is the strategy that is
the heartbeat of all your outcomes."

Awareness

This is the difference between ignorance and enlightenment in all our lives. Look at some of the monstrous leaders and their outdated and narrow perspectives. Do you actually think they have spent even one day with a coach to be able to surrender to themselves and actually show the beauty of their vulnerabilities? Instead, they stay in disempowerment and make every effort to feed only their narrow perspectives, but claim their position through wealth and positioning to further their narrow cause. They don't live their truth, and so all their efforts are powered by destructive agendas instead of inclusion, unity, and the power of freedom.

Some of the mass problems we have witnessed in the world of destructive leaders is their lack of awareness or ignorance of the good. That good can be so much greater for everyone, so why are we feeding the egos of such people? That good can be more powerful and can give them the attention they crave in such a dysfunctional and autocratic way. Look at our teaching. Our history and stories have always had bad guys and good guys, yet we have not learnt what the hero is capable of. The hero in us is far more powerful than the villain can ever be, yet the stories of villains have always made them interesting characters, sometimes at the cost of the hero. People can be sold and influenced by that. Heroes can come across as goodies—soft and mushy. If a young boy were watching that whilst also being told that boys don't cry and that they should toughen up, what do you think the trajectory would be that he would face in his life? He may not become a villain like the ones we know, but I bet he wouldn't engage with all the soft mushy stuff, because that's laughed upon and even almost ridiculed. We are hardwired into this ridiculous and false sense of thinking and perceptions. This story needs to change. We live in a world today where there is still gender bias. However, I have witnessed and seen men up on stage talking about emotions, just as I have seen women talking about powerful leadership. It is not about swapping roles but getting balance between the two, and we have some way to go as yet in this.

I don't believe people are born evil but more that they are disempowered to be good and to do good, and instead they become conditioned and give more recognition to their destructive power, their manipulative ways, and the source of early and ongoing lack of healthy attachment and experiences of relationships with other fellow humans. It is only through the offer of unconditional love, compassion, kindness, and sincerity that we can all contribute to changing that for ourselves and then for people in the wider world.

Becoming aware of who you truly are, what your strengths are, and what you can offer to people around you and to yourself, is the key to a life of fulfillment, peace, heavenly fun, and prosperity. What you become aware of in yourself can transform you and then others; it will be like you have been given super powerful eyes to see through, so that you live a life of choice and become the driver of your destination, making valuable changes to what is needed along the way from a place of knowledge and service to you. Without true awareness and insight, you are just living blind, getting by each day in such a superficial way, with your ego in the driving seat. Any feedback given to you, you will resist—ignorance is your bliss, and the destruction of self and not knowing! This is not what you have been born to do and be; growing yourself is the ultimate purpose for your life, whatever and whenever things happen. These go toward shifts in your learning and awareness. You cannot escape it, and if you harness it earlier than later, what a gift you are to humanity.

As a coach, I have experienced so many people not living a life that they have designed for themselves and are absolutely not aware of what they need to know to change it. It's like life opens a hole and they fall into it and can't get back out. It's never too late for anyone unless you are someone who has the attitude that you know it all and that no one can help. That sounds to me like a protective strategy and one that is based in victim mode and fear. In the early stages of my coaching practice, I seemed to attract fearful and uncoachable clients who really just wanted to talk to me for free by complaining about this and that; and as all good coaches would do, I would listen to a point, after which it would just become nonsense and an unhelpful coaching experience for both parties. I got better at bottom lining in order to coach the person and what they wanted in life. Some reacted well, and some just got to the end of the session, only answering what they thought I wanted to hear, followed by a superb testimonial on the sessions, and then a text or email to say they could not afford it anymore—and sometimes nothing! This lot were not ready and may never be. There is a saying about how the teacher only appears when the student is ready to learn, or something like that.

Be ready for anything on your awareness journey—it will free you up! You can lose the baggage and re-engage with things that have been swept to one side but that you truly love. You fear your own greatness and instead choose to stay small, until you start to struggle with the force building up inside you to step up and claim your purpose. There are, of course, different degrees to this, but we all have a higher purpose than what we are trained or educated in, and it will call on you to serve it for the good of others.

Mine shrieks out at me nowadays because I have ignored or dismissed it for so long! It's become impatient, and sometimes it doesn't even give me a choice. It's like it makes decisions for me so that I have no choice but to step into it. That is scary because I have to trust and believe in it 100%, and yet I have no answers, and sometimes don't even know anything. It jolts me to wake up and clear things, and to follow only the things I love doing or being: work; people; the environment; speaking on stage to get my wisdom to the masses, to radically shake up so many outdated and set ways in healthcare, education, and leadership; and for so long, this book. Awareness is the window of opportunity to be the best and greatest, or you risk leaving your true desires on the shelf for someone else to implement and own it. Imagine how you would feel then, seeing your dream being realised by someone else? Even so, your way is unique to you, and it is just as important that you step into it as they have just done. There is always room for those wanting to do more in the world, and I am happy to share that platform with authentic people.

I know how easy it is to choose comfort and familiarity, and to even struggle over abundance and success, but my calling did not let me sit still. I became aware of it through intelligence given to me, signs if you like, through the whole of me, and what I saw outside of me—the people I was once with who have no place in my life anymore, apart from being a distant memory. To get you to touch that part that is truly powerful and has something unique and important to offer, gives me the greatest pleasure when I can draw it out of you, so that you know to share it and to change something important that defines progress and leaves a legacy in this world. Don't misunderstand what this can look and feel like. It can be all bells and whistles with big stage appearances, talking and empowering masses, as well as coming across a humble and rather understated person who relentlessly and tirelessly works magic with people. It can look very different and can be of different magnitudes. Some are really happy doing and working for someone else as an employee, but they give their best every day and are known by everyone in the community. It's not what they look like or say. It's the energy or aura they carry, and the consistency and truth they live by.

When I meet people for the first time, I quickly can get a sense of them. I can feel their defense, their lack of confidence, their need to attack, their judgement, and anxiety, and then, of course, real joy and happiness, real internal confidence, a trusting nature, and so on. It is my intuitive guide or what I sometimes call my guru. When you have access to your intuitive powers, it is difficult to put it to one side, and it's hard to sometimes articulate what your intuition says about someone, so I try not to use my head to make sense of it—it is more of a powerful feeling. I was meant to cross their path and they mine. I made a difference to them, and they made me more aware. I changed something for them, and sometimes they don't get it, that it was an idea, a contact, a story or guidance, or advice or support that got them thinking a different way, and what followed was incredible for them. The ones that were more self-aware, understood the catalyst to changing, and some who were ignorant and arrogant just talked about how incredible they are and what they have achieved, without any sense of gratitude to anyone that helped them along the way. They would not know if you stood close to them and shouted it to them. The good thing with awareness is that I use it to steer myself from people who suck out my energy and goodness. I can also tell if people are genuine or not. It's disastrous for me during business networking meetings because I can sometimes see through all the bullshit that people share, promise, and tell each other. It's an ego trip steering toward performance rather than authenticity, and I wish they knew the difference. Well, perhaps they might if they attended one of my events, but I won't hold my breath.

My message to business owners is simple: For your business to grow, you must grow first; so stop investing heaps of money into short-lived solutions focusing on how to market, run social media campaigns, etc. There are a number of people who book such courses because they think this is a solution, and in some cases, having that training is good; but that's not going to be what fuels the growth in your business. Real growth in your business comes about from real growth in you. Letting go of any self-limiting beliefs, and understanding your own values, can be the green light to exponential growth in your business and finances. In my experience, it is only when you can accept that you don't know it all, and show your vulnerability and hunger to learn about yourself, that authentic power shows up. By accepting your challenges and strengths, only then can you truly come out of yourself.

People you meet will be on a spectrum of awareness, from complete ignorance of themselves and the world, to those who are truly in the flow and just get it. Sometimes experiences can take us back a step or two, but at least we know how to move forward again rather than being stuck. That's where you get fulfillment and a reconnection to purpose—your true purpose, your desire for good, your desire to make a difference. You know that feeling; the feeling this creates in you stands out above anything else around you. It is a truly powerful and transformational energy. Now, imagine if you could have that as your compass before you go about your daily life.

The knock-on effect on your physical being—your body, every cell, the water inside you, your mind, your spirit—will be amazing. It has the capacity to lift you up from depression, anxiety, and disease. Try it.

So acknowledge who you are, speak your truth, be your truth, and get on with it. Stop wasting this lifetime you have been given. It is a true gift. Be nice, kind, generous, and work with joy every day; eat and sleep well and look after yourself. You are worthy of that.

Just look at younger kids for such evidence if you can; you see, kids know nonsense when it presents itself. They have intuitive intelligence. They don't need experience; they just know. They get up every day jumping for joy, excited at the possibilities of each new day. They are aware of their emotions and thoughts. It's so simple, and yet as adults, we try to guard them from this. We interject their innocence and intuitive wisdom with our outdated beliefs, sometimes layer on layer, until they become someone else altogether, far from their natural state, each time cutting a little bit of their true joy and truth from them.

There is a real difference between kids that live a simple and outdoorsy type of life, and kids who have every gadget and whim at their mercy. Kids from poorer countries may not have the basics, yet they are so happy and hungry for chances and opportunities, and one day the tables will turn—they will be the ones treating the illnesses of kids that have it all. My perception of richer, more industrialised countries has been reversed. To be with people in poorer countries is a joy; they live simply and in accordance to nature and what is available. They still smile and have a community feel like no other, feeling proud to be alive and humble. They are true human beings. This beats bumping into people constantly on their phones, even whilst walking or taking the baby out in a pram, or people moaning about how the government does not help them, as if everything is up to the public authorities.

For me, what is heavenly to experience in this environment, where there is poverty like you could not even imagine, is the company of people, strangers even, with beaming smiles and warmth, and the way they throw their bodies around you, just to tell you what a pleasure it is for them to have you there doing good work. They don't even once complain that they have not eaten or drunk water for a few days. It's truly humbling and such a pleasure to give them the skills so that they can rise. Actually, by contrast, what goes on for the kids that have it all is actually quite sad. Our adult world and our lack of attention to them has done this to them. They are not allowed to be kids; we want to mold them into adult ways far too young, without proper recognition, attention, and explanations. They are propelled into adult ways, at warp speed, instead of exploring, playing outside, making friends, building and taking things apart, and using their imagination. They watch Netflix 24/7, or permanently wear headphones, listening to music, because they cannot be bothered to talk to anyone. Young people today have a bad attitude on being bored, constantly filling time with stuff. When I have spoken to such kids, they say that their mum and dad are never around, unlike vulnerable villagers in Africa, India, and South America, where the children there are held by people and community, their local folk. That makes such a difference to their navigation in life and their satisfaction until they can change it. That's where their drive comes from.

So to parents whose children are easily bored, let them be instead; don't rescue them with more gadgets to keep them happy. Let them stay in that place; they themselves will find a way out creatively. Shutting them up with material things thrown at them does not work their appreciation or resilience muscle. If you decide to rescue them because it's uncomfortable for you, do yourself a favour and let them be, or you will have a lot more grief later in life. Their mental health will not thank you for it either.

We need to go back to basics and lead by example. Getting your kid an iPad at 5 years of age because you have the means to, shows more about you than it is of service to your child. Be aware of that, because it's a slippery slope.

I would say that generations are meant to become more intelligent as life becomes better for us all, and access to information is so easy through the internet and social media, but it's information that they don't really know what to do with, how to apply it, or where it fits; and without guidance, they are overwhelmed and lost. This starts a classic stress response. This can then result in sleep disorders, eating disorders, youth obesity, health allergies, food intolerances, and so on.

Take a look at your life, because it is a clue. You have time to re-balance and sort things out. Commit to learning through full awareness.

Question for you:
"Time out before you read further:
'What are you becoming more aware of about yourself
as you reach the half-way mark in this book?'"

Guiding principle:
"Awareness of self is your wisdom and passage
to your soul, spirit, and subconscious mind;
it's a powerful place to be and witness as life evolves."

Chapter principle:
"To make a start on attaining health,
or even converting and restoring it, wherever you are,
think about this for one minute. Much of life and technology has
advanced beyond our imaginations, but our bodies still want to
function at a basic level, the same way as our ancestors.
So, the best way is to put basic needs in place first."

Chapter 6
Functional Side of Your Mind, Body, and Spirit

Nutrition

There is an explosion of nutritionists and nutritional therapists all around the world, and I couldn't possibly write a book on health without looking at the simplest formula of nutrition and exercise, or could I?

Nutrition and exercise guidance and advice, albeit not always helpful, and sometimes darn confusing, has been dictated by government, holistic therapists, plant-based diet advocates, and diet regimes for many years now, and if that is what is at the heart of health, then we should all be healthy right now, but we are not. We are sicker than before—can we really pretend otherwise? Let's get away from the false illusion of what health is today. The confusion created by information overload is endless and mind boggling, and what makes me sick is that anyone, even the ones with credibility in this industry, can slate trends to justify getting themselves into an influential and stronger position. It is truly mind boggling. The frustration is that each new thing marketed—cleverly of course—just seems to be a further edition of regurgitation; and still, the end user is not in mind. It is just knowledge without actionable steps, leaving so many confused and further disconnected.

So, I am not all that confident that people are interested or listening anymore, and like fashion, can come and go; it feels like a passing trend. I cannot remember nutrition courses being so popular when I was choosing what career path to go into. It was still the hardcore subjects, like medicine and biochemistry, engineering, and law, and whilst I agree that medical courses had very little in nutrition and lifestyle, this is also becoming a trend today; and I favour that doctors need to equip themselves with appropriate knowledge to deal with a much more complex illness scenario. They then, like other holistic and health practitioners, use a balanced perspective to do their work. General knowledge on nutrition is so important, especially in cooking, but that has been taken away from classrooms, and many younger mothers simply do not know how to cook from scratch. It is a dying skill and art, and worse still, there seems to be little motivation to learn despite so much of television being devoted to food cooking shows. That is the consequence of convenient foods that can give you a meal with minimal effort. Supermarkets make a lasagna tray for the whole family; it's big enough to feed 5 or 6 people for £7.00, and all you have to do is put it in the oven for a few minutes and it's done. Boil or steam prepacked and cut vegetables, and you have a meal for 5 or 6, done in less than 40 minutes or less. That takes no effort, but read the label. There are more artificial ingredients than if you make it at home. It is the same for even premium outlets selling the same. Just because they put their perceived quality label on it, with their perceived branding, means very little when it comes to processing food that is to sit on shelves, waiting to be bought.

Therefore, seeing a nutritionist won't solve the gap in motivation here. What really matters is to upskill individuals today, for better knowledge on foods and cooking and what the source of their food is—does it grow on trees or in the ground? How many school trips are to take children to a vegetable farm? Too much about food today is about its entertainment value rather than nutritional simplicity. That also contributes to overeating and overfeeding, nurturing the obesity crisis. Human health is simple by nature; try to interrupt the processes and you will be on a downward spiral. The time has come to recreate its simple formula.

People need to understand and know about food. It does not matter where you come from or what your culture is, the elders in your family are the people to learn this from—well, at least in the Eastern culture. These are the secrets that are passed down if you could only listen with hunger for that knowledge. We need to stop being brainwashed into thinking that we don't know anything about food, by people who want us in that position because then they can build their business around the solution and charge you for it. It's classic.

I have not seen anyone that can educate without some implementation tools. So many tag coaching into their offer, but they are qualified in nutrition, not in coaching, and seeing clients across a table does not make you a coach. Implementation is the key; knowledge has no power without appropriate accountable action. The issue is something else, so harping on about what to eat and how to cook it is short-lived. Remember, I have already examined the forces that exist to make it very difficult for us all to eat more healthily and make healthier choices. By all means, learn or even re-learn basic nutritional facts and how to cook nutritional meals. Some really good independent nutritionists can give you recipes to make, which include all the good stuff, but experimentation and curiosity here will help you. You have the knowledge, really you do, but acting on it and keeping it going is the difficulty. Yes or no?

So what can we do to recreate this simple formula for nutrition?

Eat a variety of foods from all groups. Buy locally and in season, and learn to cook a few basic, simple recipes that are fresh and cost effective if you are cooking for a family. Food plate and portions advice from the government is outdated, and with the view of global health now, and so much industrialisation to our food chain, we need to make sure that most of our plates are portioned mainly with fresh vegetables, small portions of whole protein, wholegrains, small amounts of dairy, non-refined carbohydrates, and complex carbohydrates, with plenty of water through the day and evening. Go to my bonus page for foods to include every day through www.JourneyIntoRealHealth.com.

Plan your food weekly.

Make sure there is as much nutrition as is possible. Don't go by what the government says—you are not stupid—ask your body; it knows what it needs to be at optimal efficiency. Your body will tell you if it can tolerate the food you have put in it or not (as long as you keep your mind outside for a minute, because we don't want it telling you that you can tolerate pizza and coke but not green beans and peaches).

Do not overeat, and it is a good idea to leave gaps between one meal and another so that your stomach has time to be empty. Forget the psychological and conditioned cues from parent messages that said you must eat this and that and eat until you are full. That won't do today, unless you get on your knees and scrub the entire floor. They ate that way because they did not know when their next meal was coming. We don't need to feast in fear of famine or lack; there is plenty of food for the entire world today, and by overeating, you won't be helping the children and adults that are in poverty and need food.
Take the focus away from food and thoughts of food. We live in a culture that promotes food and lifestyle. Just take a look at the amount of advertising, and ask yourself what is promoted the most that you are influenced to buy soon afterward.

People are obsessed with their weight—overweight or skinny—just give it a break and get foundations of food into place first. The rest will take care of itself.

Eat mindfully and be grateful that you have food that nourishes you, even if it's a little.

If you eat well, generally this will become automatic, and once the compulsion has worn out, then you will make choices that are best for you. Forget right and wrong; there is no perfection with food choices, only moderating.

When was the last time you actually saw a single advert for fruit and vegetables on the television? Hmmm, interesting? Adverts are there to generate money and profits, and there is not much profit in good foods.

I like things simple for myself and my family, and I want the same for you. Almost everyone knows what is right for them, but because of the age of super information, we are brainwashed into not trusting what we know is right for ourselves. Keeping things simple and mindful are the foundations to build on.

Question for you:
"Ask yourself what it is that you don't know about foods
that you should or should not be eating for health."

Guiding principle:
"Simply put, knowledge and education about nutrition
is not enough; it has to have a motivating incentive
and the proper mindset first."

Exercise

Let me first make it clear: I love enterprise and innovation, and something that helps people. Everyone has to make a living of their choice, and so in the scope of personal trainers, generally most work with people who want to get to a different result for their health and fitness goals—lose weight, put on weight, or stay the same, and/or build muscle—and get fit for a reason, and it is fine to see a personal trainer for that or even join a class. Personal trainers, in essence, are fitness coaches. You know the good ones, and also the ones that will try their best to keep you long enough to protect their income, so you don't get any results despite all the tweaks being made. The problem is that most sign you up into a contract for one year, and it is very difficult to get out of it because of too many variables that can affect your success, namely they can blame you for not complying. If you can afford to keep paying out because you just enjoy the company of a personal trainer whilst you train, then that's your choice. The problem is that most day-to-day personal trainers cannot really prove results, and they have usually tried a regime on themselves. Now if they are young, and most people want personal trainers of a different age, then that's the problem. You can get hooked on a fitness promise that cannot be attained, and even if it is, it cannot be maintained.

They are brilliant when it comes to help with accountability and to make sure you exercise. The industry is known to graduate personal trainers at a very basic level. Beyond that, they really do lack the experience and knowledge that it may take to make a difference to you. So, just as I advocate choosing a proven and good coach, I would ask the same of personal trainers and any other fitness professionals. Ask for their qualification and what that actually means—what are the demographics of their clientele?

For most, having a personal trainer is a luxury, as is even going to the gym, but exercise on a daily basis is essential for the bigger picture of health and wellbeing. This includes movement that gets your heart rate up, and movement and strength work that tones your muscles all over. If there is a combination of this, preferably outdoors, then this would be good for you all round.

Human bodies are not designed for the gym training environment, but today, with the absence of people working outside for good periods of time—pulling, digging, stretching and walking, carrying water or stone from one end to another, or on a farm—it is the modern-day compromise. That is the type of exercise we are designed for. It's natural and intuitive, and uses most of the muscle groups we have; and if we can do it on different terrains, that again is very beneficial. I am so glad to hear of news that there are some trainers who only work outside, getting their clients to shift logs or using a farming environment to pull and move things, rather than the convenience of man-made machinery that does most of the work for you.

So get outside more, and combine uphill, downhill, and flat surfaces to walk on. Vary your pace with slow movement and fast movement, until you can feel your heart pumping. Then slow it down again and then speed it up again, like high intensity interval training. Pack some things into a back pack, like a brick, bags of sugar, or bottles of water, and carry them around with you whilst you exercise. Use tree trunks to lean against and do presses. I mean, you can get so creative and have fun at the same time, without feeling the stress of having a one-hour window to get to the gym, do a workout, and then get back home; and it's especially helpful if you have been cooped up inside your work environment with no natural light, as it is in many offices today.

We are designed to be outdoors in nature, absorbing the - microbiome and allowing natural light in. It is the rise of the sun and the sunset of an evening that is our natural rhythm and body clock.

You become your own personal trainer, and as you make it a goal for every day, you can add something else after that, or create a walking and exercise route yourself. Local communities need to walk more. I was completing this book during the Covid-19 pandemic and lock down, and it was a pleasure to see people in my neighbourhood that I did not even know existed. They were walking in twos, in the nearby fields just by where I live. It was wonderful to see, and even after a few weeks, they looked better for it. I noticed that a few of them, who I don't think exercised and moved at all, suddenly started to walk straighter and faster. Even during Christmas, in my younger days, and because we were quite new and ethnic in this neighbourhood, Christmas lunch, for many around us that celebrated it, was followed with a walk with their family. Now at Christmas time, I don't see anyone doing that, and I still live in the same neighbourhood. Christmas Day is instead ghost-like, and most are physically affected by too much food, sugar, and unhealthy processed fatty foods and alcohol. We are our own worst enemies, aren't we?

Anyway, by all means, play sports and join classes and gyms, but make moving through walking your everyday goal.

Walking, as I have suggested, is better for the joints and condition of your body, and as long as you eat nutritionally well, it is the simple key to health through nutrition and exercise.

This can be done individually or in groups, which gives us the social needs that so many rely on when they join classes or the local gym.

Start with 20 minutes each day, for a month, and see what happens and how you feel. If you miss one, don't worry; this is about a long-term habit. It will not serve you if you persecute yourself for not doing it one day. Be compassionate with yourself.

There are so many opportunities to move your body, but instead, just as in the convenience food culture, we are adapting to a lazier culture when it comes to movement. We can go to the local shop by car, which is a 5-minute walk, and we look for the parking space that is as near to the entrance of the shop. It is really not helping us, but we can give ourselves so many mini opportunities to counter sedentary lifestyles. Even if we just stretch and move on the spot, it is better than just sitting on the couch. We are given so many opportunities to get away from sedentary lifestyles.

Whatever you choose for yourself, the important thing is that you enjoy it and do it consistently. If you are battling and regularly witness yourself talking yourself out of exercise, it means you may not enjoy it or have not understood the benefits of doing it for yourself.

Once you do, commit to it, and make it as regular as brushing your teeth.

Question for you:
"How can you simplify exercise for yourself, which gets you moving a little more throughout the day, rather than carving time out only to go to the gym—can you involve nature in any way?"

Guiding principle:
"Nutrition and exercise are simple—very simple—and there is nothing you don't know about them and their benefits; maybe you just have to want health enough!"

Self-Development and Continued Learning

I am a great believer of and really champion personal development. Of course, I do; I coach, after all, and it is only through the shift created through new learning and insight that we can truly own ourselves and live in our truth. Just go look at social media or even a book shop, and go to the self-development section; it is full of books and knowledge, written through an individual perspective on life, on everything and anything. These kinds of books are exploding into our world today. People from across our planet are searching for truth and meaning to their lives, to find a way to lessen their burden, and to find love, happiness, and fulfillment. People seem broken, and it propels them to this journey of searching. This has to be a good thing, but let me tell you that this stage in the world drama cycle has been already predicted. Today, the world—it's light and its darkness—is exactly where it is meant to be. People are tired and fed up, and there is much bad in our world, but this will continue whilst the torchbearers that guide people to light, are gathering pace to return the world back to its former glory.

When it came to my profession and longing to make a difference, I was helped to choose coaching, but not just ordinary coaching. It is true that my livelihood depends on the number of quality clients, but it is also a way of life where I can still learn and evolve, so that I can give my best by getting out of the way, managing myself in the process, and acting as a vessel in which to carry out the work I do. That's when I can be transformational. It can be tiring and awesome at the same time, and I never really understood my gift to humanity until recently. It is as if I connect to the wisdom that comes from a source that I can't see, and it is so much in service to other human beings. When I help them align with their dreams and desires that have sometimes been buried for years, which come out and show themselves again like a shining light so that they have a clear path on which to walk, and when they heal and are back to love and kindness and unity for themselves and others, it is an extraordinary experience. I am so proud of my ability as it has a spiritual dimension that I wasn't aware of at the start of my coaching, and perhaps this is the reason that I do not entertain bogus coaches that are only in it for the money and testimonials. This added dimension even surprises me when it is in action. It is a hidden force that I cannot understand or estimate, and I don't have to. I trust it and surrender to it and our partnership so that I can do the amazing work that I do for other human beings in need.

I take my gift responsibly but sometimes have fallen out of love with it—it can feel burdensome. But throughout my life, I have noticed one thing: that whoever crosses my path has always found their way, sometimes even if it has cost me mine. I used to seek why this injustice was so, until I got that it is my gift, and seeing someone else rise and fulfill their potential and success is my blessing. I had to make peace with that and really surrender to it. I know my purpose is bigger than I could ever know fully or even accept fully, but this place is perfect.

I know that many of my coaching colleagues feel the same, and we have sat and debated about other people that call themselves coaches but are not bound by ethics and authenticity, or even a genuine desire and unconditional interest in helping another person live their best life. These "bogus" coaches may seem well equipped enough in the first instance, but once you start working with them, you will understand that they lack important skills. Their first stumbling block is the necessary awareness or self-development in themselves, which is vital to manage themselves and help their clients in a progressive and open way. Coaching is an ever-evolving process and does not have a start point or even a destiny. "Dancing in the moment," as my training calls it, is all we have, so celebrate where you are and where you have come from—it is absolutely fine.

Coaches are not perfect; they are human and are sometimes trying to cope with what life is throwing at them, but it is about managing that when it comes to the client relationship, and maintaining yourself to their service is so important. It makes you more intelligent and wiser compared to the ones that carry an ego around with them because they can't be seen as an imposter. That kind of person who maintains they know best for their client, shows cracks soon enough as they become stuck and attached only to their agenda. That is to protect themselves, but if they can lead the conversation and discovery for their clients, then this allows the client to do most of the work, and to discover themselves fully. Sometimes it is touching a very difficult emotion with them. Not everyone can do that.

These bogus coaches can hide behind this illusion, crippling the richness and the depth and breadth of the coaching experience for the client.

It is true that each one of us will live a different life, and we will react to the same circumstances differently, with individual and personal outcomes that may be good, bad, or both. I could not elicit a richer coaching experience for any of my clients, without personal development myself, as long as I am continually interfacing with all kinds of people, cultures, faiths, and ages.

Being mindful and aware of yourself, including surrendering to your vulnerabilities, allows you to impact others, as well as to know their impact on you, and to manage that and not have it interfere in your ability to coach. This is a way you experience life fully and deeply, and the impact that it has is truly mind blowing. I know that coaching this way will change our world; it will prevent the collision course for disaster, the trajectory we humans are on with ourselves and our planet.

The problem about life in general is that we think all that happens to us is just that, and if you are lucky enough, life is so good, with very little trouble and strife, that you don't need to develop personally. And perhaps for a small number, whose lives hit them hard much earlier on, they learnt lessons fast enough to understand what journey they needed to be on, and as a result, their lives are great today. But it still does not stop them from evolving or being kind, or having businesses that look after their people, staff, and customers, in a socially responsible way.

But for the majority, what brings people to embrace learning and new perspectives is when they continue to have some troubles in life— some relationship disharmony, experience of bereavement, sickness, imminent death, redundancy or mental illness, stress, and so on. Only then do people want to change their ways, because that feeling of doom is so difficult for people to endure that they are either told to see a counsellor to work through their troubles, or to simply buck up and pull their socks up. In some other cultures, they pretend that everything is okay, and the family would never get help from an outsider, keeping troubles secretive.

Look at how mental health or suicide amongst men has been such a taboo subject; yet today, it has been highlighted so much more, and the general acceptance is that one needs to talk about it and to get help—to "man up" is to talk. In reality, though, how many do it?

It is very rare that I will get a call from someone whose life is exactly how they desire, and they just want to maintain it or grow themselves even more, perhaps spiritually. I want that to be different; it takes both kinds of scenarios to have a balance of wisdom, innocence, and even ignorance. When things are good, great even, it's still good to have a coach by your side every now and again. I hope this status quo changes, because self-development continues despite our material lives being great.

My vision is to position self-development and awareness at the beginning, not just when your business is falling apart and you can't feed your family. Keep learning even in good times. We simply don't spend time doing this anymore, and not in a way that is consistent. Celebrations are about celebrating with prosecco and chocolate, and bad times to be hidden from the rest of the world, with vulnerability being a sign of weakness instead of inherent strength.

Additionally, being aware, asking questions to go deeper into yourself, takes your brain on a creative journey, which has been shown to add years to your brain's life and functionality. This deeper sense of self is a must. This form of personal development and awareness is so connecting and so universal that it makes me shiver just seeing that space for all of us.

You will see how mental and physical health improves.

The human collective, when authentic and true, is so very powerful.

Learn about yourself. Get your kids to become aware of who they are becoming and what they are about; ask questions, be curious, get creative with your brain and mental health, and read books. Every situation and circumstance gives us all an opportunity to learn. Be open to that, and life will blossom; you will build resilience and problem-solving skills like never before.

Let it be known that it is only the perception of fear—which is false—that will stop you from becoming aware and then being able to do something about it. If there is something you know but want to continue denying it, it will come out anyway; so do yourself a favour and get it out into the open. Sort it out and learn from it, and move forward.

Please visit www.JourneyIntoRealHealth.com for an extra piece on being awareness.

Question for you:
"How much do you really know about yourself?"

Guiding principle:
"There are no coincidences in your life or in any life,
just opportunities and presentations in many formats that
give you a chance to learn, re-learn, and be grateful.
You impact someone else as they impact you."

Your Spirit – Forgotten in Life and Health

This is not about having a religious spin, but whilst we touch on religion, I know that I was religious yet had a broken spirit, and that was so troublesome and caused me much upset when it came to my health.

I have trained in a coaching model that in my opinion is the best because it is guided by intuitive natural forces. Sometimes my experience and that of my colleagues, who have also trained with me, was to see people who seemed to have it all but still felt empty. They still felt a yearning for meaning, and that their material success was no longer enough; their drive for life had changed, and they didn't know what it was. They would be going to their different faith meetups, in churches or in temples, but nothing they heard there quite did it either. As I am always up for a challenge and am also really curious, I wanted to work with them. It is true that "lack" can be a power source for "drive," that brings you to living your dreams and goals. There are some people that have everything in life secure and sorted, yet they feel that they don't belong, and there is a feeling that things are not in balance, even empty and amiss, and there is a disconnection.

Far from the well-known imposter syndrome, they described it as a depth of feeling that is difficult to isolate and speak about. It is a heavy feeling without any real thoughts.

Not being able to deal with it or fix it with material possessions as they are used to, it weighs heavy on their entire health.

Could it be their spirit? That also important part of you, which is the spirit or consciousness, doesn't always get a look in. You can be religious yet not connected to your own spiritual path. Many people are kind, help others in need, and are affiliated to various charities; they are grateful and mindful at times, and they are all round good people. They attributed all their personal gains, wealth, material assets, relationships, and children to their faith, yet there was an invisible force missing from the way they felt. It was indeed a contradiction.

The spiritual dimension is not about praying or going to your faith groups; it is a much deeper dimension, invisible to the naked eye, because it is a feeling that connects us to our source. Without this inclusion of your overall health and wellbeing awareness, it is difficult to balance key components for oneself, which is body and mind and spirit. It was only the coaching model I trained in that gave me the skills to help people in this place. It is not a place of lack but a place of immense calling forth, something when it becomes apparent cannot stay silent, no matter what you distract yourself with. It is an ache in your heart and belly–two of the seven fascinating energy chakras.

As a CTI coach, my role is to intuitively seek imbalances on these three areas, in a way that works within the whole self. It's tricky and works best when people can be completely authentic and open. In that environment, magic happens.

Although quite complex, your spirit is your journey as a human being, from birth to death and beyond. The time given to you in between birth and physical death is the magical opportunity you have been given. It is what is important, what gives your life meaning and purpose, from a place that is bigger than you are, and it is about learning to live enlightened, and managing your mind. I love my culture for that, and when I wanted to learn more about the spiritual dimension, I found that there is so much knowledge on this and what makes us truly happy.

It is true that when we are born, most of us have a life mapped out for us by our parents and family members. We can then adapt under that framework, depending on how close or far we stray from it, but essentially it is on the same path. We don't know that we don't know what has meaning for us and what our life is all about. For some, it is to be a leader; and for others, it is to be a change maker for a huge purpose that shapes mankind in a big way. And for others, it is to have a simple functional life, to stay at home and bring up your children or be the community person that acts as the glue that holds things together. For the most part, we don't live out our true potential and our true lives until we come to that juncture when we realise what we are here for.

The celebrity status of the millionaires, who have done something big for the world with their time or finances, and the media reporting how they have helped a school in Africa, and how they were once poor, is getting to be a cliché. I get the fact that there are some who have undoubtedly had to deal with real challenges and have succeeded in turning things around. They did well for themselves and their loved ones, and there are some incredibly inspiring and honest individuals out there, and the fact that they help people in ways that are close to their heart, encompasses their spirit on its journey, but it is media bias I am against, and the ignorant who read it and encourage it. You see, the world is not just made up of millionaires and celebrities; in fact, they represent a smallest portion but can influence the majority due to their publicity. The world is a mix of normal, common people, of all cultures and faiths, with different skill sets and different reasons to be alive at this time. But for so many others who don't have wealth or money behind them, whose spirits are centred and attuned to stay in their village and help everyone, this bias sends wrong messages. No one admires them in the media or even shares what they do, and this injustice can send ripple effects because of comparisons and the feeling of not being good enough. Now, luckily, those wonderful men and women who make an extraordinary difference and are happiest in the simplest ways, don't have social media channels to compare or upset themselves; they are shielded, and frankly they just don't care about being found or pumped up in the media. They do it because they offer themselves from the heart. The worry is not so much for them, but it's the ones that are and do extraordinary things in their homes or communities, even our young, who do have social media channels, that are affected adversely. Look at this as one source for declining mental health.

I guess, for me, having lived in Africa in my childhood, and playing with a mix of children from affluent families, as well as with the poorest children, I did know what I was blessed with, which was my health, energy, vitality, curiosity, and great family and friends, and my wonderful parents who taught me so much more than they could ever imagine. But being children, we knew nothing of discrimination in any form. It was not always through words but by actions that I learnt and noticed things, which became, in time, my values and morals, which have stood the test of time and all the ups and downs that I have faced throughout my life. This innocence, as a child growing up in Africa, taught me that as a human being I am no different than other human beings—we are from the same mold, but life's circumstances can forge differences and opportunities, of which I can make work for me and someone else if I use it wisely and with heart.

I remember, and it still is not known to my parents even today, that I packed some extra food at lunch times for my friends who did not have much, and I gave it to them to eat, with absolute delight, after which I returned to eat mine with my parents and sister at our table. I had plenty and was so fortunate that my upbringing was one of charity and gratitude. I witnessed my parents being like that, as well as all their friends and colleagues. I witnessed how my father looked after our dog, and also Juma, who stayed with us from his young childhood days to help around the house. He had no other family. I remember my mum teaching him to cook, and he became a spectacular cook. My dad used to travel, and always asked him what he wanted, if anything. My father had hoped he would say shirts, because Juma did not much care that he wore torn shirts. He had a stash of new ones in the cupboard, which my dad had bought for him in the hope that one day he may just wear a new one! In reality, he asked for only one thing—cigarettes. Juma would have one in the evening when he was alone and before his bedtime. That was his simple luxury. Can you imagine what I would say to him today? That was his form of heaven, along with his simple dinner made of Tanzanian bread and what we had that day.

As a child, I knew of no social boundaries or discrimination. These ordinary yet extraordinary people served others with love and friendship, sharing and kindness, and laughter and joy, yet no one tells of their stories. I guess maybe I should understand the draw I have for people who are underdogs—a bit like me, I guess. I can't ever see the media being interested in these people. They don't have quite the same addiction as celebrities, who crave attention, profiling, and greater wealth. Even when giving a homeless person a cup of coffee, they need to have their phones out to take a picture, to tell the world what a great deed they have done.

Whoever you are, wherever you come from, whatever your teachings are, remember to signify and uphold what is sincerely important to you, what drives you, and what your purpose on that matter is. Your overall health will thank you for it, and your reason for living, truly living, will sky rocket.

Question for you:
"Are you in tune with your spiritual health?"

Guiding principle:
"Live your life with forgiveness, kindness, compassion, and love—
that is the universal language of humanity, not just for people that
are in your life in a role, but for every living being—and that will
make your spirit happy, connected, and full of joy."

We Are Whole

This now brings me to this point at this juncture in this book. We are whole and must do and be with that, as it's an overarching and protective quality. Let's work with what we are as a whole—mind, body, and spirit, the whole one energy—we need to understand its power. Take a minute to understand what makes you whole. Can you imagine what is possible for us and to each other from this place? This is where our higher self resides. When this energy field is balanced and connected, can you imagine what is possible for us and how everything can work in balance and synergy? It is about joining the dots.

As a coach, this is what I aspire to for all of you; it is to bring to everything and everyone in our lives the optimum body, mentality, and spiritual dimensions in what we do and become.

Our heads are connected to our bodies, and our spirit energy dimension runs through the whole part of us. Just look at the number of spiritual leaders that do chakra work and help us unblock the unseen channels—the energy fields that help us be our best and higher selves, that part that is enlightened and aware. When we are open to that, only then can we share the gift of life and living in a connected way with others, and in turn impact them to do the same.

With a focus on health, which I hope by now has changed some of your perspectives on what health truly means, aside from the superficiality of only tackling it through food and exercise, how much of our health care directives only tackle our health piecemeal? That then makes it like a home project, doing one room at a time, when the opportunity, money, or time exists at that set point. By the time it comes to getting and completing the whole home, the rooms that you started with are again falling apart, and hence we start again. Integrated health cannot and should not be tackled that way. It is only through working on the whole of you that you will understand and feel its impact on your life in a positive, sustainable way.

Today's healthcare is set up for management, not on the true focus of wellness at any given time and moment. We get passed on from one person to another, where we see multiple people for one concern, without anyone ever joining the dots. That's where you come in, because I don't want you to wait for that. It may never come, but you have the intellect to own your health just the way you desire. Don't complain, don't seek too much information, and don't blame anyone, including yourself!

All systems that are from outside work against the fact that we are whole; but from within, you can make it your core principle in today's world. Well, that's if you want health in a more sustainable, healing, and energising way. There is no other way.

Our mind, body, and spirit does not run like a business, but businesses can be whole. Organisations, in this way, can benefit people so that they are not actioning relentless tasks but are being given fulfillment and meaning, whilst creating much needed stimulation, without exhaustion, allowing the freedom of working the way that they are naturally good at, without micro management and cloning practices. Businesses of the future must have heart as its core principle.

Again, education is another area where our spirits are broken from a system that is so unnatural to the way we learn and progress, because like other businesses, it has become a tick box exercise and far removed from the intention it had set, which was to educate and inspire our minds to achieve their potential and be in love with learning. Instead, kids over the age of 16 are being told to stay in education when they don't want to, so that parents can claim benefits and then further get their kids to have financial help for food, travel, and other costs. How will this ever help those kids? So many actually know how to work the flawed system, and some of my teacher friends tell me how rude these kids actually are—they have no respect for themselves or anyone else, but those same people detest the real poverty on the streets in other countries. They take it as their right for hand me downs.

I admire any government who steps in to help genuinely needy citizens, but where they give, they pinch from somewhere else. It has not actually affected them personally.

So, as taxpayers, we can instead instill charity and kindness, skills of resilience, and a state of gratitude in our children. Can you imagine how that would be? I can see much of the world becoming more balanced, equal, and kinder if we educate that way. There will always be wealth, and in some cases, some will have more than others. We have to accept that, but this is not at all about wealth in the pounds and dollars way. The wealth of wholeness in our lives is the future.

The wealth of unity and oneness is the only way forward, and the quicker we can educate our young this way, the quicker prejudice, racism, discrimination, violence, gender bias and inequality, and even the demise of our planet, will cease.

Question for you:
"Think about it; when do you make important decisions
from your whole self?"

Guiding principle:
"It is when life is lived from here, that it seeks a peaceful and
uplifting balance of bliss. You are whole; don't forget that."

Chapter principle:
"Join the dots between your functional side of body, mind, and spirit. Health in its best form is only when all these three features are in balance. Eat good, highly nutritional food, not just empty calories. Do exercise that you enjoy so that you aren't finding yourself making excuses, and connect your higher self wholly."

What Comes Naturally to You

Chapter 7
Learn from Children or
Your Childlike Part of You

Intuitive Know-How

We are born in tune with ourselves: our needs, desires, emotions, and thoughts. At the start, it is a primal need to just survive at the hands of carers, mums, and dads.

At birth, we have everything just right for our utmost survival. Our minds are open to learn basics, and then evolve to learning more complex patterns, but we are ready nevertheless. That is the greatest gift in life: to learn, to develop, and then continue learning.

We can create in ourselves to inspire, educate, and equalise our world that we share together. I have mindfully been watching children, studying mine and also those of others as well as the insight from my own childhood memories. For some reason, I am drawn to them, and many would say that they are drawn to me as well. In fact, personally, I have more young fans than I do people of my age. I have learnt more about myself and the world around me through them and my own children as they develop into grounded young adults, than I have through adults, and what becomes less of them and more about their ego. I don't want to learn from someone's ego—no thanks.

Children have a direct connection to their hearts and minds, and by observing them, we too can be connected to our hearts and minds.

They have a pure form of wisdom, with equal measure of purity and innocence, which is so endearing, and yet we strive in our adult ways to take that away from them too soon, by exposing them to adult ways and behaviours. Schools do not allow them to be children. They hurry that process, cripple their curiosity, reduce their time with nature, and set them on a course to become puppets and disconnected from their authentic nature.

Just watch them today if you can, and do it without any preconceived ideas of who they are and what they do; just watch as if they can't see you there. You will find moments of pure magic. It's one of the most beautiful things you will witness. They may be playing or otherwise engaged in something, but they are also just "being," and I am not necessarily talking about two-year-olds but the whole spectrum of childhood years. It shows us peace, happiness, and joy. Now, also think of the last time you felt this in yourself, what you were doing, who you were with, and where.

The shame of getting older is that they start to communicate from outside influences and teachings—yours, their teachers, their friends, and of course, from information across the web. What happens in time is that they stop listening to their intuition and the knowledge that comes from within; the connection to their internal self depletes because their ego takes over and sometimes overrides what is the truth. This intuition and inner strength that children show in their earlier years is quite amazing, and this is exactly what we need to harness and preserve for our lives as adults. In today's teenagers and adults, when their ego minds are pressed to play, the old recordings and stubborn outdated beliefs of others take precedence over their own voices of strength and knowing—the inner master voice is diminished to silence in time. Think of all the times that you used this ego to make your decisions, when your intuition or childlike voice had said something quite different, only for you to realise that the wisdom within knew what was best a few months down the line.

What we do as adults is to overthink, whilst kids don't do this—they are more connected to simplicity and the joy in life. When we overthink, we lose that pure connection between our minds, our bodies, and spirits—our hearts. I have been at the centre of children losing their mother to cancer, or their father to wars, and I can't tell you how amazing their resilience is, because their grief and acceptance is pure. If you were able to clear that and just be with that emotion for a while, you will find your strength and resilience, just as kids do, and healing is more authentic and comes from within. I am not saying that it's easy on any account, but there are less of the consequences that grief and not healing properly can create further down the line. Furthermore, being connected to all your emotions is important, and many answers that we seek for ourselves in life and health are there. Look at what information they give you; don't be afraid or feel guilty. Notice them and learn. Allow yourself to feel the full spectrum of emotions, not just the happy ones.

Their intuition is their greatest asset, and this is how they navigate their emotions and behaviours. Remember that the survival instinct is quite high when they are babies and young children, and that's generally their compass to navigate who and what they are comfortable and safe with, because they are not independent enough to fend for themselves completely. Having such innocent wisdom does not mean they are mature for their age. Wisdom that is pure and integrated into the fabric of your being does not just come with age or experience. It is there right from the beginning, a template waiting to be written on. That's why it is so important to let kids be just that, and that kind of pure intuitive wisdom is there with them forever, even though the access to it becomes a little more challenging as we take on layers of crap in our daily living. It is not good to allow children to grow up well before their time.

I know, in some instances, there is no choice but to rely on children. In some cases, they become the carers, and the strength and resilience shown by these children is remarkable. They can be looking after a parent or younger siblings that have health and addiction issues. All the inherent skills that children have, which are vital to live their lives, is something that is still within us even as we transform into adults. There is a childlike part of us even as adults. This childlike part of you has access to the same skills you had as a child: purity, innocence, wisdom, intuition, joy, and creativity.

The question is, how can protecting and accessing those natural intuitive skills help you in your own health and wellbeing needs?

If you think about it, health and wellbeing is a basic need, and we have systems in place that automatically come into play when needed. It encompasses sleep, eating, social interaction, communication, learning, stimulation in both body and mind, thirst, and withdrawal needs (when attention goes suddenly as a way of protecting against over-stimulation).

Now compare all that to our grown-up world. At what level do we automatically look after these elements? My guess is: very inconsistently!

Why?

This need is interrupted by a false need based in ego. When was the last time you felt hungry physically and decided to delay feeding yourself for hour and hours, not just because you happened to be in a meeting and didn't want to be seen chomping on an apple out of your bag, but even soon after the meeting? Maybe then? Maybe not, because you have booked yourself into another meeting? When was the last time you felt sleepy at 10 p.m. but insisted on watching a film till midnight, and when you felt thirsty but had something to eat instead?

We regularly override some basic cues on a daily basis, so who are we to blame our own illness, through these consequences, on something else or someone else? Remember, the fingers are pointing back at you!

Are we good at saying yes and no when it's needed? Do we sacrifice our needs over the needs of others?

Our natural intuitive instincts are still there to serve us if we can open ourselves to them as children do. These mechanisms serve to bring us into balance—a better state of being—it's all about balance and harmony rather than extreme measures of coping.

We need our bodies in homeostasis, our thoughts in balance, and our actions appropriate and in alignment. You see, when kids are hungry, they will eat; when they don't get food, you know about it. In contrast, when we are hungry and we are not able to eat, we don't stomp around crying; we hold out until we can't anymore. That is not to be celebrated; its plain stupid! Do that a few times and you will start to change your unique and individual patterns that were there to serve you. We live and work in a world that expresses general ways rather than unique ways, but I hold out on strategies that can include both. We are brilliant at adapting, but we don't need to over-adapt!

So, the first rule is to be careful in your communication with little ones, and that little kid in you needs to be cared for throughout life. Don't overrule them when they say truthfully that they are full and can't eat anymore, even if they have left their greens. Say that's fine, because you trust that they know their appetite; in fact, praise them to have listened to their body's intelligence, telling them that they are full enough and have to stop, even if they have not finished their vegetables. But let them see you eat yours with great enjoyment. Just don't overeat and overfill your plates.

We have children and then society trains us to train them to become adults well before their time. This is wrong. I am all for good and decent, safe behaviour, especially whilst in public; and again, it comes back to the values of the family in terms of what and when things get taught, but when it comes to their own health and wellbeing, they know! Not because they have read loads of books like you, or spoken to your friends and followed trends, but because they have their own intuition of what is right and wrong for them at that stage. They are mindful and make decisions at a given moment, and they have the right to say no, even to the most desirable meal cooked for them. Just watch, and don't overrule them by making it about you being right. It's a massive ask, I know, and you will feel guilty or even angry and very uncomfortable, and even start the internal conversations with yourself around whether you are even cut out to be a parent, but this is your ego in play again, rather than your natural desire for protection and nurturing. Take a step back if you find that you are in a quandary between multiple voices. Children are not designed to starve themselves. Please don't override that natural cue for less or more.

I remember very clearly, during the early years of my firstborn, when I convinced myself that she was not eating enough, and I made sure she finished everything that I thought were the right portions for her. Luckily, the portions I gave her were not as big as other new mothers gave to their babies and toddlers, but it was nevertheless too much for her. Even the extra one last spoonful was too much, and she used to tell me in her way, usually by blocking the spoonful coming her way, by turning her face. Or if I did win and get the spoonful in her mouth, she would spew it back out, much to my frustration! I sometimes listened to what she was trying to say, depending on my mood and degree of tiredness, but her reactions and strategy were consistent, depending on if she wanted more or less. She was communicating in her own way each time, but I was not listening; and even if I noticed her actions, I would overrule them with my agenda.

Then, one day, I decided to stop listening to my health visitor's advice and all the other new mummies, and tried to connect with my child and her communication from within, rather than a hit-and-miss approach and a process of elimination that most parents have to grapple with when they are novices at parenting. When I did this, and got to really know her and her personality and her sincere intuitive guidance for herself, even though neither of us knew what that meant at that time, the battle of wills came to an end, and mealtimes with her became so much more harmonious and joyous. It was actually liberating. I now know that my attachment to feeding was only confused with a cultural dimension: Nurturing by feeding is a big thing in the Indian culture, and a lot hangs on that aspect in terms of the sheer satisfaction you feel when you feed your loved ones, close friends, and visitors. My child was not refusing to eat; she was refusing to overeat. There is a difference, and it can be as close as crossing the line with half a spoonful extra to what is required. Today's obesity epidemic has its roots in overfeeding, not just in the type of food that gets eaten. You can be obese by eating too much of the healthy stuff too! People eat too much of anything today, and when physical cues and natural intuition are ignored, they create a problem. Learn to trust your own knowledge. You are your own master.

Thankfully, I was self-aware enough to realise the potential harm this overfeeding could have created physically and psychologically for the both of us, albeit done with the most loving intention—it can be turned into damage and destruction. Thankfully, all my children are healthy and happy, with their intuition intact, which they regularly use to make important decisions that are right for themselves. Our attachment together is healthy and sustainable for life. That's an achievement in itself.

So it is important to learn to manage ourselves throughout our lives, and how and when we communicate to our young, especially when we don't know or care about the full impact it may have later on. Parenting today is trickier because we have let in so much bias. I have never had any problems with my children loving healthy foods—they have such a healthy relationship with it, and they are mindful of foods on the so-called unhealthy lists as well, but they eat those too, when they fancy it.

You will make mistakes, and that is okay as long as you rectify them as quickly as you become aware of them. The big mistake is when you know something is wrong and ignore it—that is stupidity, and you will know how easy it is to be trapped there. There is no perfect place, but balance is not about being perfect. So stop chasing the unachievable, and instead go for moderation, mindfulness, and balance for yourself and others.

The way that outside influence can infiltrate your mindset is given with this example, which resulted in me doing what I mentioned earlier, trying to get my kid to eat too much. The need to overfeed my child came about by the health visitor who insisted on telling me: "She is not growing... you are not feeding her correctly... she is too little ...." Note here that she was NOT underweight, and she had no health issues at all! This was all about comparative theory, and not related to an ethnic baby weight, which by tradition is smaller at birth than the Western comparative.

In my mind, it was all about "not enough." My friends' kids ate like monsters, so I tried consistently to overfeed my baby, and she fought me every time. Thank goodness, she did, because I could no longer handle "the battle" at the feeding table. I gave in, and looked at her and thought that she was not only healthy but was full of energy. Her skin was baby soft, clean, and she had no allergies. She loved vegetables and fruit, and was eating well enough—she was just a personality who knew what she liked and didn't like, and she knew confidently what was enough for her. Today, she is a grown woman, healthy and whole.

We are not born to abuse ourselves or to go hungry, and it is only when I trusted this that I became more peaceful, stopped comparing myself and my baby to others, and I did the job of any good mindful parent who just wanted the best for their child. I became one with them through my own childlike state within, and this resulted in the pure joy of having them and seeing them develop and grow rather than the stress that most parents are under. I went on to have another three healthy, energetic children. My brood is all grown up, and they are amazing, if I say so myself and they are not perfect and certainly do not fit into archaic societal norms. They are lively and progressive.

The other side of the parenting spectrum are anxious parents whose language is always about watching what you eat, micromanaging every single ingredient. This is so counterproductive and becomes a self-fulfilling prophecy. They are also disconnected from their own intuition, and instead are operating from a place of fear and criticism. That's their parent-like ego.

The best way to be with it is to relax a little and be mindful rather than anxious; manage your mind and emotions. Eat a little bit of what you love, let your children eat a little bit of what they like, and trust them. Don't deny it for yourself, or you may start a mechanism of craving and then binging.

It is such a pity that the world we live in today is so judging of so many things, and parenting is one of them. I am confident, assertive, and educated, but when I had my children, I felt judged, as if people were saying that I was not a good enough mother. I remember that feeling so well today. Let's learn instead to be mindful, and respect that each one of us is unique, and know intuitively and intellectually what is right for us in any given moment; and if we can start with that with our younger children, and we allow ourselves to nurture that, then there is the gift, with wings.

One exception to this is if you see your child putting their fingers in a socket or running on the road! Intervene immediately!

Question for you:
"When or where has your intuition guided you,
and on reflection, can you thank it now?"

Guiding principle:
"Your intuition is your inner compass for the outside world."

Natural Hunger

Hunger is a state we feel when our bodies are in need of basic functional nutrition. This is called physical hunger. The basis of functional nutrition is to keep us alive, and so that our bodies, at the cellular level, have energy for all the differing functions we experience and use, including the copious amounts of repair work our bodies have to do to keep us alive and well.

We have an exemplary flight or fright response, which serves us in times of danger and for our survival on Earth, and we need to be able to access instant energy in case we are running from a tiger, like we may have done way before in our primitive lives. This allows for the lungs, heart, and blood to serve us in this feat, helped by the response of some stress hormones. Today, of course, we don't run from tigers, but we perceive fear, lack, and stress, and are in a constant state of lifestyle stress. This means that our stress response continues and has no way of actually switching off properly, and so we end up with stress related illnesses, as well as other severe metabolic changes and illnesses. The tigers of today could be the failing of finances, unsuccessful life management, work environment, dysfunctional home life, trauma, and loneliness, as well as failing relationships, as some examples. It is strongly founded that overindulging in highly sugary and fatty foods, alcohol, and smoking are lifestyle coping responses to this. This is actually counterintuitive to what we are meant to be eating for. We therefore can use these coping mechanisms in order to give ourselves some respite from these stresses; and what happens in time is that we weave a whole web of behaviours, friendships, and communication around this, which eventually becomes an identity. You may know of a friend or an acquaintance who is lots of fun but drinks ten pints at every pub visit—everyone loves him but himself.

So let's look at it from a child's perspective and how they eat when they need to, because they know when they are truly hungry and when they are not hungry. You can put any of their favourite things in front of them and they will leave it, because they eat for physical and functional reasons. They don't know that is what they are doing, and if they get told constantly to stop eating, or to eat constantly, they will lose that important cue. They will get confused, and this is the case for our children of today; they eat through greed and boredom, and that's when they overeat on sugar. They don't have to have any illness at this time to tell you that this has to change or they will be ill later on in life, and perhaps even become overweight.

I always remember one particular scene in my life, when my children were all young and still had the wonder of Easter eggs. I would hide some eggs around the house and get them all to look for them, and then put them in a basket for them all to share. These were typically smaller ones but with colourful wrappers to make it exciting for them to find, and also for them to view them all together in a communal basket. What I noticed was that no matter how much of their favourite chocolate was left over, they all ate it at a good pace, and to my surprise, eggs were always left over, which many times I threw in the bin, or at times I would finish them myself—more the latter! I hated waste then, and loved chocolate—the combination of those triggers was dangerous for me.

Over the years, I noticed the same patterns every year. They all had a way of rationing their eggs according to their physical hunger. It would pain me more to see chocolate eggs left or half eaten. I had to work really hard not to finish them, and what I noticed was a voice that said to me, "Don't waste them; you spent money on them, and it's rude to waste food." That was the first time I noticed the "finish" cue! And luckily, from earlier experiences with the health visitor, I learned that these were my issues, my self-talk, which I did not want to pass on. They were outdated, and the world did not need more human dustbins. I also learned that they were more excited about the eggs and the game than they were about the chocolate itself. It was the experience associated with it that was their delight.

When looking at physical hunger, what you will also find is that some children can go without food for long periods of time (like 4 hours or so), and some are constantly needing top-ups and snacks (every 2 hours), which means eating small portions frequently. Whatever the natural pattern is for them, its fine; please don't overrule it.

It is really important to keep to regularity with what you feed your body, and also in terms of timing, and keep this going as best as you can throughout your life. There is the right degree of satiety when you are in a natural pattern. The level of satisfaction is higher, and eating nutrient dense foods, and eating them regularly and in a natural timely rhythm, will help you keep alert and well, and your metabolism fired up.

This will also protect you against establishing emotional eating conditioning—a type of "false" hunger that we see more of today. It is complex and ends up with a person mismanaging their thoughts and emotions, and therefore their behaviours with food and drink. The compulsion to eat something is huge and overwhelming, but it is not nutritional and functional eating. Emotional hunger does lead to overeating and therefore putting on weight, which today is very common amongst our adult population and, sadly, becoming a concern in our children. Please do visit www.JourneyIntoHealth.com for an extra bonus on Emotional Hunger- it's not what you eat but why you eat.

As human beings of all ages, we all need to be challenged, and so the right balance of stimulation and rest keeps this type of hunger satisfied; in fact, when you feed it food and drink, these fail to satisfy it, and that's because it's not the real reason to need food. Nothing quite satisfies it, so we just keeping filling our tummies until we can't physically get anymore in. Our stomachs are maxed out and we can feel the pain, which some people celebrate—can you believe it?! I can't believe it but can understand it. Most that do this, eat and drink mindlessly; they are distracted and in their heads, which is why I advise, when you eat, to do just that and nothing else. Yes, round the table you can talk at a good pace between spoonfuls of food and sips of water or drinks, but that's it—no phones, no television, no thought of all the work you still need to do—just attentive eating and enjoying your food. Jump out of your head and pay attention to your eating mechanism, including digestion.

A proven way to stop this emotional eating or hunger from taking hold, is not to reward with food or gestures with food, but instead to eat only for nutritional purpose, thinking of what your body needs in order for it to be in its best form, and if you have something missing in your life that you are craving, go get it. This could be giving love and receiving it, sharing love and intimacy, being authentic and generous, having gratitude daily for all your blessings, and working toward your dreams and desires and toward fulfillment. When this, for example, is lacking or is inconsistent in its presence, that's when a never-ending feeding graze takes shape, resulting in diminishing health. Please watch this pattern in your young. They are now eating like adults, predisposed and in their head, whereas their natural patterns are disrupted through modern living. My upcoming book, *Ice Cream or Green Beans*, covers aspects of this to help children stay healthy and functional, and close to their natural patterns.

Natural physical hunger is patient and gradual, so eat only when hungry, which is easier to say with so many of us trapped in other people's timings and work. If your cue is to eat at 10 in the morning, then kids are either in the classroom or you are at work. This inflexible way of eating when appropriate cues are surfacing can be difficult to manage, and unless you can have the freedom to choose your schedule, the best thing is to do it as near to that time as is possible. Remember, it does not have to be a meal, but it needs to be nutritionally high in content to really feed you and to nourish you. We have to come away from the conditioning that feeding means a plateful; it can be a boiled egg with some crudités made of fruit and vegetables, and with a fresh-made dip of hummus, or a sweet, homemade flapjack full of seeds and dried fruit, which are naturally sweet. The choices are infinite. We need to get better at planning this and being creative with good but simple food. It can be done despite budget and time restrictions. You have to make a decision and have intent, that's all.

Continue to be curious when you feed your body with food and drink. What is tolerated is digested easily and is a cue that your body can process this food. If you get a tummy ache or feel low in energy even after eating food, it is not being tolerated. Please do not ignore these simple signs and guidance from your body if you want to stay healthy and decrease possible inflammation in the future through deteriorating gut health.

If you are obsessed with foods that you cannot tolerate, please stop. When are you mostly happy with food, and when are you not? What triggers you into drinking alcohol or eating things that are unhealthy despite your health and wellness boundaries and agreements? What happens next?

The problem we have today is that little children, who have amazing radar for this unnecessary eating, eventually get overruled by parents or authority, and they can no longer navigate what is right for them. They are getting complex messages to eat and to eat more. There is 24-hour access to food today. We live in an obesogenic environment, and the call for food plays on the minds of all of us. Children need more guidance, but they will only get the necessary guidance if the mixed messages cease and they see their parents and relatives doing the same. You can teach them the right things and the wrong things, but you are still teaching them. Take that seriously and without giving criticism or judgement. Lead by example, and lead from there.

What they are taught, in a way that is empowering and explained with love, at the early stage, will impact them and serve them very well. We owe them to practice and master good health, and the human relationship with food has to be a healthy, balanced, and a rational one.

Question for you:
"Take a minute and think about what your pattern
for natural physiological hunger is."

Guiding principle:
"We are all different, but most of us sit in boxes for the day,
churning out stuff and worryingly ignoring our own physiological
cues, one of them being natural physical hunger, which is when
your body wants nutrition, not a Coke or a bar of chocolate. It has
work to do, and feeding it empty calories is an assault on it."

Thirst

Let's eat less food and drink more water—all of us. For any food that you can eat less of than you are at the moment, and replace with plain water, the better.

So how?

Well, firstly, there may be some confusion between thirst and hunger signals. Most of us are dehydrated, and considering that most of our body is composed of water and cellular fluid, where many cellular transactions take place in water, we really must consider becoming well-hydrated at all times. Getting water in when we first wake up, throughout the day, and into the evening before we go to sleep, to last all throughout the day and whilst asleep, is crucial. We don't really think it is necessary because our thirst signals send us to fizzy drinks or water in plastic bottles with sweeteners and flavours, which are not going to hydrate us. Drinking something else is not quite like drinking good, pure, clean and filtered water to really hydrate us, and I guarantee you will feel so different when your body becomes accustomed to being hydrated properly. Our body stores food but it cannot store water, even though the majority of the body's composition is fluid, so replacing it regularly is so important to maintain health and mental alertness.

Today's craze on energy drinks that so many are on, is such a concern. Why would you need an energy hit just to do a regular day's work? What's the real problem here? What's lacking that causes you to lack energy?

In our busy lives, we have very little time to drink enough water to keep us adequately hydrated. I know from experience that working in corporate organisations, retail, banking, or manufacturing, gives very little time provided for drinking water. We certainly don't do enough in schools; our young are going without water for 6 hours of their day most days, and are instead drinking juices laden with sugar and artificial chemicals at lunch break. This is a disaster for their health and concentration, and may be attributable to why so many may then go on to buy energy drinks with their pocket money.

Getting to meetings, making the day importantly productive and successful, teaching curriculum, and making every second count in our business, steers us away from water, in fear that we will need inconvenient toilet stops, and that is the reason to not drink enough water. It's laughable that such complex and intelligent human beings can make stupid reasons up to ignore their biological and biochemical makeup. Well, maybe it's time to stop selling yourself short, and to think about what your body needs and wants. I have heard of call centre organisations where staff are not allowed to even carry a water bottle with them because they don't want orders and sales to suffer, and some have told me that they can go for long periods of time without a drop of water so that they do not interrupt the chain of sales orders. I would walk out of any company that puts profits over basic human needs and actively discourages it. It makes me so angry that people cannot even voice their concerns in fear of consequences and authoritarian disciplinarians.

Don't they know that firstly you can actually sip water for long periods of time before your bladder actually needs emptying, and then don't they know that dehydration can cause a lack of concentration and mental focus and alertness? Healthy, happy, and capable staff leads to better profits. Such companies are examples of incompetent managers and leadership. We need to respect that drinking water and eating, and having adequate breaks, preferably in fresh air, is a basic need and not a performance indicator!

We live in an era of stress, chronic fatigue and disease, and decreasing mental clarity and proficiency, and we are becoming inefficient in our work, which costs the economy vast amounts of money anyway. Why is the model for health not changing?

I find it bizarre that in some past and current schools in the UK, and certainly one that my children went to, drinking water was not encouraged because it was a "disruptive" practice, thus sending messages to the children that their wellbeing and basic needs are not important. It is also important to note that most teachers there have a high sickness statistic! Now my kids regularly bring such observations home to discuss with me, and whereas I am mindful of the fact that teachers do have to get through the academic criteria, and that there are undoubtedly some kids who will disrupt for the sake of it, they are in the minority.

I have been in the health and wellness business long enough to know the impact of dehydration on all of us, and on children in particular, around their focusing and concentration levels. This is how it went in one of my children's schools: They started out with allowing named bottles in the back of the room, which they could have whenever they wanted, but that got stopped because of one disruptive student who was doing this only because he could not sit still and had to work on his attention gauge. Instead of dealing with his issue and supporting him more, the problem became the water bottles, so all 32 children had to go without because of one kid. Can you imagine the impact on that kid? It is often the case that a minority—and in this case, one kid—is able to disrupt something for all his fellow class mates. That would either go to his head or it would make him embarrassed enough to give him other repercussions. The policy change to having no water, because of him, was beyond any logic to me.

Why are educational institutions supporting and actively discouraging health in our little ones? Surely someone from the science department should have a say. They would, I hope, have studied simple biology.

The fact that they got water only at breaks and lunch, resulted in the water filler taps (very limited numbers by the way for the number of children and staff in school) being swarmed by kids, all trying to get some water. This resulting chaos was often seen by the lunch time supervisor, who had only one focus: to keep the noise down and get them out of the door for playtime, often ignoring the pleas from kids that they were thirsty, and then quickly shutting the door and pointing a finger, saying, "Out, now." They, of course, go and make themselves a nice cup of coffee. Where is the love here?

Perhaps it is missing because education is free, after all, and children and their families need to count their lucky stars to have a place at school. Is that the primary factor?

How are we letting this type of education environment sustain the army camp orders? The frustrating thing is that you won't see this rubbish during an Ofsted visit, because only the best behaviour is seen. I have worked in a school environment, so I know how totally fabricated this is.

It used to wind me up big time to see such false collusion from staff at every level of the school.

Today, we have an education system full of people like this—all protecting their backs—and it lacks great or even good leadership from every individual that has any authority. Lack of integrity becomes the new norm. Is there any wonder we are short of skills required for the workplace, when these educational environments are full of too many stupid rules made through lack of respect for students, the very people they are meant to serve to the fullest potential? We moan about problems on our streets, and even though our kids spend most of their days at school, it is the parents that get blamed for such behaviour problems.

It is a collective problem rooted in our society, and the school environment has a massive impact on kids' mental and emotional health. Sometimes the school environment is the only saviour for some individuals who have such massive challenges at home. The schooling years are a massive responsibility for education and all the people in it, and I have yet to meet the modern teacher who is able to cope with the responsibility they have to their students, and have the necessary mix of skills to champion, motivate, inspire, and challenge for their best potential. Education, as it is today, is not attracting able candidates with the right motivation for such a responsibility to their learners. Yes, they can talk a good story, but in reality, it is no longer good enough. But then I see the argument that this type of army camp is fantastic training to then go off to the corporate world, because they get it there too. Do I sound just a little unhappy here? It is my and many other parents' experience in the last ten years, and to date and only getting worse, with crippling funding, lower quality teachers, and stress. This does not bode well for a healthy environment for many, and certainly does not make it an inspiring environment, which is what learning has to be around.

The resulting outcome is that we do not live and work in environments congruent with health and wellness, because we don't speak it, show it, or even practice it. It is just not important enough, and that's the collective problem. We instead concentrate and are so taken in by productivity and selfish, agenda-driven incentives that we cannot even come up for a breath.

Whilst there are organisations and schools that do pay attention to wellbeing, it is not consistent, and again, a tick-in-the-box exercise. I cannot be happy with such standards, as are many other parents, but as a coach, I am even troubled by it. The statistics for home educated children is rising steeply because children or parents, or both, cannot face the schooling environment, and the failing teaching and health standards.

What happens over a considerably short timeline is that the kids get fed up with this, find it too difficult to challenge their teachers and speak up for themselves, and then they just go without. The teachers, on the other hand, think that they have managed the situation with success, when actually the kids' needs are put aside and go underground.

What happens when we prioritise other things instead of what our bodies need, like simple water and food, is that we, children and adults, stop listening to our bodies. Many adults who now don't drink the suggested amount of water for their weight, or eat good nutritionally complete food, have learned to override the basic signal for nourishment, because that meeting is just more important, when actually it takes no time to have a water bottle and sip on it all day long to keep hydrated, and to have a prepared, healthy packed lunch, which can be eaten in less than 15 minutes. If you can't even take 15 minutes out to eat, then you need to look at your daily life and see what you are prioritising instead, and why.

It is bizarre that I have to make a point of this. I want to keep children and adults knowing the basic and real cues for physical hunger and thirst, and then the difference between that as well, knowing and then prioritising these over other things that are filling their to-do task list. Knowing when you are thirsty and not hungry will also help you to not pile the pounds on. Many, these days, are so dehydrated that they mistake it for hunger and end up feeding themselves with food and not water. Let's observe and learn this from them, and encourage them to trust and act on what they know of themselves, even if they see the detention room or get a demerit at the age of 15 in school.

So, no matter where you are right now, drink some good plain, and if possible, filtered water; drink it in a glass and keep that going every day for the next 30 days, and you will see a massive shift to better energy and focus. Work on drinking at least 2 litres per day, as an adult portion, to start with. Drink it in small quantities and throughout the day, rather than a big lot in one go and then leave too much of a gap; and always drink to your thirst, so that you may drink more, and that's okay.

The quality of our water in tap form is another debate, and so is the water in plastic bottles. So, wherever possible, drink from a pure copper vase or BPA free beaker, so that the water is not leached with toxins from plastic, and it has a chance to actually hydrate you. Tea, coffee, and alcohol are all toxins and have a diuretic effect; they dehydrate you, so please keep them to a minimum.

Your chance to support any children yourself is to drink water as your main drink per day. Leave drinks like pop and fizzy drinks, which have additives, unseen sugars, E-numbers, and artificial ingredients. If you have to have them, keep them to an absolute minimum.

There are so many apps available that can help you with drinking water on a daily basis, so do what you need to do to make sure that you are drinking water throughout the day. Work on identifying your signals for thirst, and the difference between that and hunger, so that you feed your body the appropriate fuel at the appropriate time with full awareness. Let children get into a habit of drinking water whenever they ask for it. Please don't tell them that they will fill their tummy too much for them to have food. Water is as important as appropriate food, if not more.

I would get my children to drink water in the morning before they ate breakfast, and to fill their water bottles, and then if they could, to refill them through the day if at school or college (sadly, hidden from the teacher's gaze!), and after school. They tended to sip water throughout the evening until about 40 minutes before bedtime. They would wake early and with energy, with no headaches or pain, and they were not ravenous and gulping down anything sugar-laden in their path.

If they missed breakfast, I didn't fuss as long as I knew they had water and that they had a pack up for their first break at 10 a.m., which was usually when they were hungry anyway. As they grew up, they in fact started missing breakfast as they slept in a bit more, but having the break from the night before, to perhaps 10 a.m., was a good thing; and today, many of the intermittent fasting principles work on this time frame. For adults, that first meal of the day could even be 12 midday, from 8 p.m. the night before as the last meal. It allows for autophagy in the body, which is an incredible and physiological process of the body regulating organs, and detoxification and energy balance.

On days when I don't have the necessary water, or my children don't, I know the difference it makes to the quality of our health, concentration, and energy.

The point here is to learn the difference between thirst signals and hunger signals. Children will identify the differences quite simply. We need to retrain our brains to understand the difference if lost or confused.

If you are not sure of the difference between hunger and thirst for yourself, then whenever you think you're thirsty, have some water and see what happens, and also do the same for hunger. If that feeling subsides and is satisfied for long enough, then it was thirst; if not, then it may be hunger of some sort, although it may not be physical hunger but instead emotional hunger, so check with yourself first before you give your body what it does not ask for.

Question for you:
"What is your daily water intake?"

Guiding principle:
"Set a routine to drink water throughout the day; you may be able to go without water, but your body will really struggle—good restorative health starts from as basic as this."

Need for Attention

This is another fundamental and basic need that we have as humans. I touched upon it earlier. When we respond to this in an appropriate way, it forms a good basis of a good healthy attachment to oneself and others. We need to be recognised, and when we are younger we get a lot of it through touching, kissing, and cuddling. We develop skills and get through certain milestones, which are also recognised and celebrated. Kids are so touchy-feely, and this is how they make sense of things.

You may notice that you need attention, and when you don't get it in a way that is yearned for and meant, sincerely and congruently of course, you feel a sort of lack. It feels like a bit of a void—sadness even. If this continues for a period of time, we do start to become lost. This genuine need does not ever go away within you, because there is a childlike part of you that is very mindful of this, so from time to time, it will assert itself and creep up on you to answer to it in appropriate ways. You have to become good at articulating this primal desire. It could be about existence, or fulfillment, self-care, or self-love, or about giving and receiving, or being free-spirited and joyous, as most children are born to be.

I like to call this type of attention recognition or touch hunger, and it can be very positive and desirable for living life to your full potential. Without this positive reinforcement in our lives, and it being such a life-giving need, we may turn to getting attention in a negative way. The need for any attention, whether that be positive or negative, is rewarded when it comes to our survival and recognition. We want to keep it as supportive and positive as we can, and therefore we need to learn to become mindful of the clues and signals, and when our moods and emotions are telling us that our recognition tank is depleted or near empty.

So it is important to know what you pay attention to and what you ignore. That is perhaps more about game-playing, which is hankering for attention from a place of a victim mindset, looking for ways to lead to unhelpful affirmations about yourself.

Many people have said to me that when people do recognise them, it does not feel genuine or sincere, and that may be the case. There are people who throw about compliments for the sake of doing that, but even if you have one person who wholeheartedly loves and cherishes you, and that can include yourself, that is enough for now. Sometimes it is because you don't think enough of yourself in a sincere, loving way. Perhaps you believe that you don't deserve or have not done anything life changing for yourself or others that may have helped you fall back in love with yourself. Perhaps you are playing small and have only danced to that tune.

Think about when you were a child, and you took your first steps or read for the first time. How joyful were your parents or caregivers, and how much attention did you receive on every early developmental milestone? It probably came as happy smiles and loud clapping, and cuddles and joyful announcements on what you had achieved. It was normal, and most parents know that, but the relief and pride in you was being recognised albeit conditionally at every developmental milestone, and lots of it nevertheless, celebrated in such a way that it must have felt extraordinary to you and them. You were you, a precious, living, breathing little person, and they thought of you with incredible hopes and dreams. That then was unconditional love.

As we grow up, that form of recognition changes or even dies down, because we are told to toughen up, be strong, shut up, and show no emotion, as that shows weakness or excitability, which are not favourable in wider society. The kind of attention, as you grow older, is more through words and gestures with certain tones and actions. So much now becomes more about conditional rewards, achieving exam success, or taking piano lessons and being able to pass that exam, and so on. It is about how thin or fat you are, how good you look, what clothes you wear, and who you hang around with, especially if they happen to be popular. That is society's judgements, and it can be kind as well as cruel. Lack of kindness can erode self-esteem, so it is very important to surround yourself with people who truly care about you, just as long as you remember that not one person can be everything to you—that's too big an ask.

We do what we do, and live our lives according to our chosen paths, but let me tell you that the current phenomenon is to not recognise yourself until you are amazing, have conquered something, or have become a millionaire after living on scraps. The way we measure success is at fault and the way we focus on success is all wrong. We are all, at some time in our lives, called forth to show our extraordinary selves, but we all have so much pressure to prove it first, before anyone can take us seriously. That in itself simply loses my interest. It is like we all have to prove ourselves, and without that, we are nothing. I think the greatest strength is sharing the journey in real time as it happens, when you actually don't know where it leads to—that is what we need more of. It's about taking people on a journey with you, not just giving them your answers. Being able to stay with the unknown mess and uncontrolled unpredictability of life and the journey we are all on individually, collectively, and uniquely, has more excitement and strength than something that is marketed and fabricated.

We have to restore unconditional love and respect that we have for everyone, including ourselves. I remember first going onto social media and, after a few years, I started realising how dreadful it made me feel looking at other people's lives and comparing mine to theirs, because I was in a place where I did not have a husband or money to go on holidays, or just could not post photos of myself with the children—not because our relationship was rubbish, but they were not interested in it. I don't come from a social media era, and I keep my views and engagement with it as realistic as it can be. I like to mix it up. My children were happy to take photos with me, but they just did not want it ending up on Facebook. That's surprising as they have all grown up with the explosion in social media. I stand reassured, I have to say! I resorted to the fact that my kids were just different and did not feel the compulsion to show the world what they were up to every second, just to frame everything in the name of content.

Such great wisdom, even at their age!

I guess I am still a little old fashioned in that I really, really enjoy simple things, like sitting on the couch with my family and talking, hugging, playing games, and laughing, even though my kids do tend to make silly videos of me and now laugh at that too. My life behind the scenes seems complete, so there is hardly any motivation to capture everything just for content, but I also know the value in social media, and there are ways I can make good use for it. Surely good things, meaningful things, showing good in people, talent, and wisdom can be shared, and social media is one of the greatest platforms to do this with. The problem is that there is so much information that sometimes it can get lost, or like me, I can switch off to it. I guess I have learnt that it is not about me but the impact it may have on others; perhaps others need that level of sharing. It has to be part of a mix.

It is good to remember that not everything that gets shared will be good for you. It leads to information overload and, every now and again, it has the capacity to unnerve me and make me feel inadequate. It gives me the fear of being left behind, when in reality I know I still lead in many areas of my life, and it can do that for you if you are stuck in a void, wondering which direction to take and what's next.

How much content gets posted just astounds me. I would not have enough content in a lifetime to keep up with some that post every few minutes, with shots of themselves with this person or that. Now, I know that some content is repurposed and used again and again in new, fresh, and evolving ways. Even if I tried, I have very little time to post or even schedule posts, so yes, it's my weakness, and I would gladly let someone else take care of this side of me. I have to engage with it and embrace it if I am to succeed in getting my message out there.

But for now, and for you and for your health, switch your mobile devices off for at least one day, for the entire day, and spend time in the sunshine and enjoy your loved one attentively. The worse thing is to pretend to be attentive and then multi task, which includes swiping your phone every few seconds and pretending you are listening. Be like little children in awe of the day ahead, and leave social media behind for a while. Don't click every moment with a camera; if you pursue keeping your brain and memory healthy, that is the most powerful camera you have.

Capture it there, the full experience. You will also help your brain stay healthy and well throughout your life. It will service you by keeping you sharp and able to take on information easily and openly.

There are exceptional people all over the world who will never get the chance of speaking on stage, or even know how to self-promote themselves, and in essence, they don't need that.

One of my biggest frustrations with business people today is this ethos of good PR, except there is a fine line between having a real heart for it and being sincere, compared to the inauthenticity of having a connection to a charity for marketing purposes. The charity doesn't care what purpose you do it for—it's fundraising. There are many conversations with business people that I have had that made me really frustrated, because they sometimes can't even recollect that they have been associated with a certain charity, or what work they have done; and when asked, not to interrogate but to be genuinely interested in the good work they did there, it transpired that it was a clever PR illusion. They paid money to be associated with their charity of choice, and despite the social media content, in person, they come across as confused and can't really speak about it. I find that so strange, but then, maybe not. There are some genuine business people who do brand by association and who can talk about it, and even teach it, because it has helped them get out there and help more people in their mission.

So be careful what your branding says about you, because it needs to be consistent on any platform; and also be careful to not be taken in by inauthenticity and false PR. In those companies, people are interested in one thing: themselves! Getting hooked on such can cost you your mental and emotional health.

Grow your radar, like children naturally have, and know the lies from the truth.

I know it's hard being authentic and genuine; the world as it is today steps over that as having real value. The ordinary as extraordinary is not seen by people. If you are so much of a giver, the world looks upon you with skepticism; they have come to not trust that without thinking that you can't give without asking for anything back. It's true; people find it difficult to trust, and people don't recognise goodness when it presents itself. Truth is diminishing today, and so it is expected that most people misjudge a genuine person unless that person is also authentic and genuine so it is easier to recognise each other and these people will support you in anything you want to change or even disrupt to bring greater good to your world. Others do not like change.

Notice how children have no way of discriminating or holding boundaries. They remain versatile, adaptable, and resilient whilst any changes are going on, and they support each other. They have no reason to judge anyone, and they trust their heart. They ask for attention when they need it. All this can go "pop" if the adult is not centred and grounded in the same way. Time and time again, I have witnessed parents betray their children's heart and innocent wisdom by telling them to judge, to discriminate, to love a certain way, and to be wary of people that are different. That's where discrimination and racism is taught, even without knowing it. The list of opportunity is endless.

Let's look at the other end of the age spectrum: older people. Here is an example of what today's convenient and at times lonely culture means to them, and why the need for attention is so important. An old lady that lived a few houses down from me usually went to the local village to get her shopping—mainly bread, and meat from her local butchers, of which there are now not many in local high streets. She usually gets on the bus, and we need to recognise her for her age, her health, and wisdom, and how she is still integral to the very fabric that makes our society loving, diverse, and inclusive. When old people feel like they are an inconvenience to society, and a burden, they die! Never make them feel that way, ever! She looked ordinary, but she never outsold her kindness for anything. Knowing how hard she worked all her life, she still managed to smile at every one that passed her. In my eyes, that makes her extraordinary. She may never make it in the news because she is not quite 100 years and is ordinary, but she is independent and healthy, which also does not make interesting news. Instead, the news can continue reporting on evil and terrible division, giving it centre stage, not only on our home screens but on our minds.

Why do we need to know this over other good news? I am not saying that reporting every old woman buying bread and getting on the bus herself and smiling at everyone, and showing unsurpassed kindness to her neighbours, needs to be on the news, but then again why not? Maybe it's time to give ordinary people doing extraordinary things the significance they deserve and others like her, through our own frame of reference as news to us, it may bring a smile of gratitude to us, and increase our appreciation of ordinary people being extraordinary.

I think that there needs to be a fundamental paradigm shift on what is right even in the news being reported—I have a choice: I don't watch it—I don't need to have it reported to me to know what is going on with our people and planet. I see the consequences.

Recognition and adequate need for attention will exist; decipher what the real need is, and if it's genuine, then give it the recognition it deserves and make it count. It must be sincere. With badly behaved children, give them attention on what they do well, and you will see the bad behaviour disappear. It's like starving a fire: Don't give it fuel. Anything that is bad or does not serve you or anyone else, especially if such behaviours are associated with getting attention and recognition, don't reward it.

In addition, give yourself recognition and attention for everything you do, no matter how small and ordinary, like everyday things like cooking meals, cleaning the house, having the lawn done, fixing the lights, getting a great customer review, or just spending time with each other, or choosing to say no so that you can do something more meaningful and important with your loved ones—and then go and recognise five other people, for who they are, not only for what they do or don't do.

Let me give you an example of how crucial it is to give recognition correctly when attention is asked for, and not reward bad behaviour. During group coaching, I had one lady in the group who was deliberately disruptive. Her triggers were not all obvious at the start, but then when she displayed unhelpful actions both to herself and to the other members of her group, it seemed obvious and there was a pattern. She was wired to act, react, and behave in a very childlike manner, which usually got the groups attention. She was sabotaging the ways and achievement of others in the group as well as her own, and grappling for the lead position in the group, only displaying what other's perceived as her own self-importance.

For a while, the others in her group resented her for being there, which meant that she dug her heels in even more. The environment started to become toxic and began to feel uncomfortable, and I felt that it would have been the easiest thing for her to be asked to leave, but that would not break her patterns. So I opened up the group for sharing, and courageously and openly asked her to speak about what was going on for her so that she could explain her ways. She gained a lot of attention in her childhood from doing naughty things, and she explained that she never felt enough love from her parents, who only voiced their opinions and judgements when she did something naughty. So what was rewarded were the actions she took as a child that caused her to gain attention, like hurting her siblings, being a fussy eater during family meals, breaking things in the house, and being labelled as "naughty," and then being punished of course, by being sent to her room or locked out in the garden for a few minutes.

Regrettably, her parents did not know what to do with her, calling her names like "needy," and telling her that she was just an "attention seeker," and commanding everyone publicly to "ignore her." She was regularly sent to her room for isolation whilst her siblings were able to stay downstairs and play games with mum and dad. This disruption and unruliness continued at school, and teachers also branded her with similar titles. So many opportunities were missed to meet her needs. It is no fault of anyone as parents or teachers, because no one understood her basic and emotional needs, and furthermore, what the consequences of not meeting them would eventually be over time!

Keri was not proud of herself, and deep down she craved love and attention unconditionally rather than just get attention when she did things wrong, but in the perceived absence of love, she learned how to exist on drawing attention to herself—any attention—from ways that were disruptive and created a guaranteed response from her parents. She often said that she could not help it, and this behaviour played out in different locations, with different people, throughout her life. It was only until she was not judged and was given positive reinforcement that she began to change. She was 55 years old when she came to me. She spent the greater part of her life in this disruptive way. If I had told her to leave the group, which was what she was expecting, it would have been like her parents sending her to her room whilst everyone else goes ahead and gets on with things. It was by opening her up to a simple gesture and space being held for her that she was able to help herself. Many people may say that I should have acted with the majority needs in mind, which was to get rid of her in order to keep the others, but I chose to allow learning for the whole group, because the majority were blind themselves. She had more awareness than the others. They all learned that one can make a change for many.

Luckily, today, she is a much happier person and has many loving people in her life, and she is working on her relationship with her parents, who she blames even though they could not have known. In such cases, the downward spiral starts young, and that is why I pioneer health and wellbeing in all of us, in a holistic, engaged way, from day one. The integration of physical, mental, and spiritual health is the key. Working on only one aspect is not enough, but starting to work on one with the full intention of learning about the others, will be wonderful for you. The principles and topics in this book are signposts—strategies if you like—to implement, starting today.

Question for you:
"Can you fully think of a time when you felt recognised
for who you are or for what you did, and can you experience
the feeling again in its entirety?"

Guiding principle:
"Always pay careful attention to what is being asked for."

Rewards and Treats

We all need rewarding. The best reward is to be healthy all your life. Actually, it's more than a reward; it's the master of rewards, which makes it a true gift. This way, you have the potential to live life to its fullest, with great joy and harmony, and with your values and purpose intact and integrated into your being and doing. If you have everything but your health, this will cause a massive deficit because life has to be adapted, interrupted, and intervened. Having your health so that you are able to do what you want in life, and making choices of living that would otherwise not even be contemplated, is a gift—surely, you see that, right?

Athletes push their bodies further than we have to; their window to be the best is short-lived and crucial, and to get to the top of their game before age catches up with them. They have a small window of opportunity to get their bodies to be the best they can be, and so their training and career is centred around the only chance they have. Because they push their bodies to their limits, it is easy for them to tire easily, and they are more vulnerable to serious injuries. If they are in their prime of youth, they can heal quickly with the right interventions. Whilst they are in that window where they strive to be their best, their regime for their health has to be exceptional, and their reward is the lasting legacy they leave in their sports arena. Their medals tell their story for life, and even beyond.

We can look to be the best we can be, but that is different for everyone, because the starting point is so different. So you can never compare your health with the health of someone else. I don't think athletes can with each other either, even though their goals may be the same: to win gold for their country. We can therefore set about looking for rewards that also last a little longer; and for us to enjoy them, we need to make sure that all aspects of our health are in service to us.

What I mean about rewards lasting longer is that most will choose to celebrate with something—a meal out or a trip to the cinema, a holiday, or even a social gathering like a party. These are, of course, great rewards that are tied to achieving something, and there is a huge variance in reward choices between people and what is achieved.

Like I said, rewards are an important feature of life, but we tend to base rewards on what we did, what we achieved, and our successes in something. I want to change that dimension a little. I want you to reward yourself for just being you. I don't want you to wait until you have achieved a goal to set a reward in motion. A good mix of unconditional (being you) and conditional (what you do) rewards would work best to make you feel that you are moving forward. There cannot be rules made for rewards, because we all need to be rewarded in some way, and it can range from very simple to a huge set up, depending on what you really like and value. These rewards act as building blocks to you feeling worthy, and then you need to build layers so that, together, they are sustaining you and lasting throughout your life.

Watch the easy rewards of food and drink—this is overused today, and if you have an awkward and unhealthy relationship with food, then that can be challenging; and the other red flag is grandiose gestures, because that can build a false illusion of yourself. I know many parents who fall into this trap and then wonder why their children don't seem satisfied, always wanting more, or they simply lose their hunger for ambition.

I hear children telling me what their parents gave them for just cleaning their rooms, or have been a witness to parents who say, "Get through this term without any detention, and we will take you on holiday with us, and you can bring a friend." This is a kid who gets detention for bad behaviour at school, and the parents are a little embarrassed, so instead of finding a solution to the core problem, they tackle it with plaster therapy, an incentive, or even an emotional bribe, a common theme amongst parents who don't really know what they are doing or how to tackle the difficulty and challenges from their children.

Adults get to open a bottle of wine as a reward for just getting through a work day normally. You see, in some of these examples, a reward is more a bribe. In a world where instant gratification is the way, rewards are becoming more like gestures rather than what I am talking about. If there is a reward for getting the kids to clean their rooms for two weeks solid, I am not sure that they will do it after that without the same or similar incentives—they are not choosing to keep their rooms clean by themselves, so they don't understand the importance of that in their family. Once they do, they may do it, and you may not need to bribe them. It will get tiring, and you will run out of bribes, or the bribe will not have the same impact, so the challenging behaviour will continue and perhaps even escalate—so now what? What we need is engaged children. Too many of today's children know the deal: They get what they want too easily, and they know how to play you. I get parents telling me how they actually fear their children, not through abuse or physicality but through their emotional blackmail and manipulative tactics. Children are clever, and they will learn clever ways in order to get what they want.

Let's get that back for them, by encouraging them to be self-sufficient through the love of just having their rooms nice, clean, and tidy. It is when they do that by themselves that you reward. The timing is essential for engagement and the greater good. Rewards need to reinforce positive actions and affirmations, sincerely acknowledging them for who they are, and not only for what they do or don't do. That means you have to know them, see them, listen to them, and accept them. See only their pure form, the form that they were born with.

Recognition, as you have read, is the life-blood to our lives, and rewards are part of this process, adding structure or tangibility to that recognition.

Think of the last time you gave recognition for something or someone for just being who they are, and how that felt and how it impacted them for being acknowledged and recognised in their true form. It's when you get to your children properly, peeling off all the layers that society wants for them, and you acknowledge that it's absolutely beautiful. I bring acknowledgment to my special way of coaching and I have to say that it brings me to tears, usually with a lump in my throat, which the human being in front of me is also processing. When it lands, and they absorb it through their body and the layers of their mind, it opens their heart in such a powerful way. That's the reward that lasts way beyond anything that's ever known. It can feel like a rebirth, like a powerful white light enveloping you and holding you while you feel loved and acknowledged.

It is okay to mix this up with tangible rewards, and if meant sincerely, then there is no problem as long as you are mindful. The kind of rewards we give and expect are actually too easy to give and receive, and can be against health and wellness. So children get sweets given by their teachers. Call Centre staff teams get given a pizza on the house when their team comes out on top. Food is cheap, accessible, and easy to give out. We all love food, need it, and enjoy it, but I think we need to be really mindful about what we choose to reward with.

When I was leaving work to have my twins, I remember the feeling I had when I was given a basket of goodies for my unborn twins and for myself, which included self-pamper goodies, flowers, and books to read, and a beautiful framed picture of my team to remember them by. I truly felt the love and the effort that so many had put into to getting me something special. I am not sure, if they had just taken me out for a meal or given me some food items like cakes and sweets, if it would have had the same effect, although I would have been grateful for anything. To this day, I have the framed picture, and it brings so many great memories of my time there and makes me happy. I was only there for a year too, so it was also an acknowledgement of the positive impact I had made, and then sharing the news that I was having twins brought them into the experience with me. I think it moved a few of them!

If food has to be your thing to give and receive, then engage with healthy foods or high-quality items instead of the majority of what gets rewarded, which is crap high in sugar, starch, and processed ingredients and additives. If you want something different, think of activities, holidays, walks in nature, or just spend time out in the garden or on the sofa with that person. It is being or doing whatever gives genuine pleasure, not something that ticks the box. Nothing is worth giving unless it is meant to be given with and not through convenience or cost. Spending time with someone with all your attention is priceless. It's the attention that is the true reward to both.

Our brains know about rewards and pleasure, and quickly learns from association, which is why food can be a stubborn association to break. Arranging an activity or going to the cinema takes a bit more expense and also needs organisation and effort on your part, so it is a little trickier, but it is good to have a full spectrum of the rewards that you can experience for yourself. You know that a walk in the park or a book to read is sometimes better than fish and chips; we just have to teach our brains to feel as good about it as we do fish and chips.

I suggest a good brainstorming session on all the different things you love, and then match them to what feels right for you, in keeping with your best health and not deteriorating someone else's.

Rewards don't have to be grandiose. There are so many experiences that are delightful, and if budgets or time don't allow it, then spending some time with someone you love is a reward. Just sitting in the garden or on the sofa, or walking hand in hand out in nature, and spending time with them attentively, is one of the best rewards. Giving our time to each other, and giving it with love, lasts and builds that foundation I mentioned earlier.

I can hear people saying that altering food rewards may be challenging for some, but let me ask you if this becomes about being together or does it become about the food? I see so many couples and families who hardly talk to each other these days when they go out to eat at restaurants, not because they are unhappy but because it's all too familiar an experience. There is no novelty or surprise anymore.

My children have always preferred time with me rather than routine feeding frenzies at a restaurant. The power and focus of food is so great that it can take away so many other wonderful moments with each other. My children remember time spent cuddling in bed, far more than all the countless meals we have had together. The memories of the laughter and giggles far outweigh memories around a table in a restaurant. It is true that the emotional experience of happiness can never be forgotten, and even Alzheimer's patients, who cannot remember details of an event or person, can connect with emotion and their feelings. The joy of daily living has to be turned around on its head. Too many are set into a routine that feels mundane and trapped. Feel the joy, however little, in each moment, and live mindfully.

Question for you:
"What rewards do you give yourself and others?"

Guiding principle:
"Rewards of the right kind that are healthy and wholesome
are just as important as breathing; give yourself
a meaningful reward daily."

Emotional Intelligence

How lucky are we to feel a full spectrum of emotions; what great insight they give us. It is the feelings and vibrations from them that tell us how to think and behave in any given situation. They give us the insight when reflecting on the past. They are a window into our world of thoughts and behaviours, and all three are linked in such a way that one influences the other and is impacted in some way. It is truly amazing when we are in touch with them, and the signs we get when we are aware of our emotions can truly transform our actions.

It is so important to be in in the moment with them, and to learn how to be in tune with our true emotions. I say "true" because sometimes there are "racket emotions," which are manipulated emotions that are not congruent with the appropriate emotion—for example, laughing when you experience the death of a loved one.

We know that emotions are linked to our thoughts, and our emerging thoughts and thought patterns are linked to our fundamental core beliefs. Emotions of fear, anger, happiness, and sadness have a purpose and so cannot be affiliated to being labelled as positive or negative, but it's more the use of them and how they change your behaviours; the thoughts you have that can be more on the negative/positive loop. It's more about appropriate and inappropriate emotions. Children's emotional tool kits are unsurpassed. They are very much in tune with their feelings and, again, conditioning them to feel emotions or not to feel emotions, because of someone else's core beliefs, can be devastating in the way they end up navigating life. If you can't cry, think about who taught you that. If you can laugh again, who taught you that? Do you fear everything before you can achieve anything—who taught you that way of living?

It is again our conditioning that stops us from becoming informed of our emotions—you know that saying, "boys don't cry," and that type of banter that floods our young boys' impressionable brains when they are so young. This type of conditioning stems from beliefs of others, which seem to grow wings when a new baby comes along in the family. Some of these beliefs are very outdated, and some are appropriate, like traditions and proven ways of family life. Be very careful what you pass on. The only way to reassure yourself with passing on the right things will be your own self-learning and awareness.

It is also just as important to note that all emotions are necessary. I mean, if you were being chased by a saber-toothed tiger, then you would naturally feel fear because your thought would be that you are going to die, and you are not ready to die as yet, so the emotion and thinking patterns are appropriate for you to survive and run faster. It physically opens up your physiology to run; muscle groups are activated, you witness speed that you never knew you had, and your mouth becomes dry and your breathing fast. Your intuitive guide is at its best, and you don't ponder—you just run. Good job that!

It's essential for your survival, and it could be only a second's difference between running away, hiding, or being eaten alive. If you did not know that tigers can eat you, perhaps you may have tried to shake their paws, but because of the way survival and living is handed down, and in those days was pretty simple really, you ate when there was food, you slept, you gathered round to talk to your family, and you ran from tigers.

It doesn't matter where you are in your life right now, but having a clear understanding of your emotions is a good thing. When you lose a loved one, it is natural to feel sadness, but it is not right to feel guilty if you eat cake, like so many do; but so many, despite feeling guilty, do it again and again. That guilty feeling does not change the behaviour—have you noticed? It's like you are addicted to feeling guilty—what's at the core of that, I wonder? Who taught you to feel guilty when you eat cake? I am not encouraging you to eat cake, but I do not encourage feeling guilty after you have eaten it either. The latter is most likely a rule from someone somewhere, that cake is bad and you should not have it; hence, when you do, you feel guilty. And then you eat more of it, and then it moves along a little more on the full emotional guilt spectrum, so now you feel shame because you can't stop yourself, and you don't know what is going on. Remember, I touched on emotional eating earlier. Are there any insights here for you?

This is the problem with inconsistent and confused messages. Emotions and feelings must remain intuitive, and you must trust that the correct feelings will show up when appropriate—or are we so disconnected from ourselves that we are tampering with an intelligence system that helps us survive in the first instance and to thrive later on.

When I eat cake, as long as I choose to and have made it myself, I feel fine and happy; and because it is a mindful choice and not an action to block difficult emotions, I can stop at a few mouthfuls.

Many people that I meet and have worked with, have emotions that are confused, and many just don't want to connect with them. It is as though the softer side of them may show a crack or weakness, and it is easier to hide it away. Our emotional system is incredibly intelligent, and when connected to it, only then can you access and are able to articulate intuition—your sixth sense. So connect to your full spectrum of emotions. They will pass by—watch them, hear them, and feel them in the moment; learn to dance with them, learn to be patient with them, stay with them if you have to, and learn to dive into them—and then when you are ready, let them go, and learn something that they tell you about yourself in that moment.

We live in an era where people have become so ignorant of themselves that they are two different people: one for the outside world, and one for the world inside. Accessing emotions has rules and regulations of when they are allowed to surface, or to be shown at all, and it just makes people so inauthentic that you never get to know the real person; and don't think that just because you live with them, that you know them either, unless you are all authentic and have done work on yourselves in terms of self-discovery and awareness. If you are able to know yourself better through your emotions, you are way further than most people, and you will witness how children are naturally attracted to you.

We live in a collapsed cycle of thoughts, feelings, and behaviours and actions—how do we gain any knowledge of ourselves that way? We need to become better at knowing our minds, learning from our emotions and supporting our behaviours.

Kids do this well; it is very rare that you see a child that will not show emotions. When they cry, they tell us something; when they smile, they tell us something. When they are happy, you know; and when they are fearful, you know. They know these basic fundamentals, and they know when they need help and when they are okay on their own. They share their emotions and have no rules—it is natural to them, and they use them to navigate and communicate. It is a lot easier asking for help when you share your emotion than when you don't. People cannot read your mind, even when they try to, but they can notice your state. When was the last time you needed real help and needed to ask for it? And did you or didn't you? Or did your mind overrule your emotion and tell you to just get on with it!?

What was the thought that went through your mind when you couldn't ask for help even though you know you needed it? What was the emotion you felt?

I completely understand that sometimes not showing emotion is a protective strategy, and this can be used by many who have suffered or experienced some difficulty in their life. They mask the undealt-with emotion by either being frozen in emotion or too loose with their emotions. This is terrible for health, so what I want for you is to show up every day as genuine, dealing with things, and taking the time to understand yourself, your emotional drivers, your emotions, and what your truth is! You cannot ever influence or be anything to anyone until you can be your true self.

I know that when working with children, I want them to protect their emotional intelligence and fully own it—I must teach them what I have taught my children, which is what comes naturally to them, and to look out for how quickly emotions can be masked by experiences, after which we can make too many rules about feeling happy, feeling sad, feeling angry, and feeling fear. Let's not; there is a reason and purpose to all four emotions. Let's make use of them, and use the intelligence they give us as a valuable tool.

I remember being told not to get "excited" when something was exciting, like a holiday. This was from my grand aunty who felt that getting excited meant that it would not come true, and that I would be disappointed. So to save me from having the feeling of disappointment, she told me to stop being excited. For years, I wanted to get excited about so many things, but I was too afraid to show and feel it, in case the thing that excited me would fall apart and I would lose it.

That was so self-limiting and went against by real self. Still knowing that, even today, feeling excited about things feels wrong sometimes, and I have to make a real conscious effort to feel naturally excited when something good happens to me. It is getting easier, and as a child, of course, before that rule impacted and influenced my ways, I would have felt excited about all sorts of things—just like kids do! My aunty had passed before I could tell her my insights, and I am sure her intention was love. It was, after all, protective love for the experiences and beliefs she had built in her life, except she sabotaged her experiences with disappointment.

We don't think about what we say to people and how it can influence, but as in this example, it was passed on, and I did not know any better—why would I? This self-limitation was easily evident when I wanted to step up my game in business and wealth, because I had to get excited about the potential of it; and instead, I kept pulling myself behind the scenes, still working hard, but anything that I achieved, I did not say or tell. It was better to stay small because, that way, I could contain any excitement and not have anyone else take it away!

I have given myself that mission and purpose. That means I have to step way out of my comfort zone and claim my excitement about not only my future but the future of everyone I can impact. I have given myself permission to get really excited.

Today, I get so excited about speaking and being on stage, and this feeling lasts long enough for me to push boundaries and make a change.

People don't like when things go well for you. I was told many times that life coaching is for the weak, and that people like me are nothing more than a good Samaritan wanting money, and that there was nothing exciting about that. This was from people in the general public, on social media. There are so many ill-meaning people who would rather you suffer than have a life of abundance, opportunity, and continuous growth. Some people just don't get it, do they? With the unkind world of biased opinions, is it any wonder that adults tend to play their emotions down? It is better to fit in than stand out, right? It's easier; I get that, but the easy way plays havoc with my peace—the bubbling in my tummy doesn't rest—it wants me to step up, to challenge the darkness that is becoming the normal in the human spirit. I do and will, no matter what. I say to stand out, and that it's good to be different, to disrupt the normal and make it extraordinary instead. I don't need to take care of those unkind people—the naysayers—a different intervention will. It's not my job to change people who resist their truth so much. For my work, for you and me, it needs courage and excitement.

Question for you:
"Which emotion are you fully allowed to encounter,
and which ones do you step over and dismiss?"

Question for you:
"Which emotion are you fully allowed to encounter,
and which ones do you step over and dismiss?"

We Like to Please

This is in all of us, and we can learn how children like to please us, and when they are recognised for it, notice how happy they feel. Pleasing each other is so pivotal to sustaining a community of well- meaning and wonderful unity in people.

The need to please is very strong in children, and their behaviours are driven by this urge. It gives us tremendous feedback on who we are and how we stand in this relationship. I remember my first swimming competition after moving to the UK. It was a new school, and I was keen to do well, as did my parents wish for me. I remember that I had my eyes on my parents and family, watching their expressions as I entered the water, and after completing my win, I looked straight at them, and I saw them clapping and smiling, which was reinforcement of my belief in myself, and also of their belief in me. It was the making of a confident, happy girl. Later on, I observed the same of my younger sister. I am a big tennis fan, and I love to watch the top players competing with each other; and I notice, despite their skill and experience, that at pivotal points during their match, they can be caught looking up at their coach and their team, the people who have invested time and energy and faith, and have coached skills into those players. If the crucial point is won or lost, they still gaze at their team to feed off the messages of pleasure, encouragement, and support, and sometimes challenge. This can make a difference in keeping the player grounded and focused; whether they win or lose, the supportive belief from the team is the real deal. That goes for athletes who can feed off their supporters, so pleasing them is a crucial part—it's a natural part of being a human being, and is a win-win and is equal in its outcome. It can be a form of double recognition, and also the driver to keep going, winning for themselves and supporters, friends, and family. We almost expect it at staged events like that, and it is equally important to have it in our daily lives. There is nothing more devastating to our human spirit than wanting to please, only to get ignored or dismissed.

Nothing about giving and receiving love, if it's from the heart, is false or detrimental ever!

We also look for that moment when we want to please someone and they acknowledge it. It feels wonderful, doesn't it? When we proudly present their gifts for birthdays or Christmas, when we see their delight, it fills our hearts. We know how it feels to witness surprise presents being rejected. It's the same for children who come home with what they feel is the best picture they drew of you, and you look at it, and instead of reveling in their effort, you kind of dismiss it. They wanted you to be pleased with their effort and their masterpiece of you, but it just fizzles to nothing. Always find a common ground; there is something good in everything. Don't rush your thinking.

You know the times when your partner had made a special effort to cook you a meal, and all you did was moan about it not having enough salt, or some other complaint. Well, maybe you had a valid point, but you should have known how deflated your partner felt, even though I am sure they can take the feedback. I believe there is a way to say everything without conscious ill effect.

We like to please, and as long as you are mindful of that for yourself and others, then there is health and wellness in that. Take note of when the balance tips toward pleasing people because you don't believe in yourself enough, and you crave being liked because you are desperate to be liked. That's a different state of being. Healthy pleasing and unhealthy craving are different human states to be in. The latter is based on desperation and fear, and even if you do get acknowledgement and recognition in this state, you will still try harder and harder because you don't believe you are deserving of love and kindness—you don't trust it. This will erode that relationship and your health; it's a very hard thing to sustain, and too much to ask the other person to endure.

Then there are some who are also people pleasers, who talk, make polite gestures, talk of collaboration, show that they are interested in your world, say they will introduce you to this and that, are understanding, empathetic, and make promises, and make you feel excited for something you talked about, only for it to fizzle out. They asked you to get in touch with them, and when you did, there was nothing there—they had fallen off the Earth's axis, and you couldn't get in touch—they outrightly ignored you! That says more about them than you. Let them be, and make peace with it; it will help your mental health for sure. I meet people in business like that all the time, and as much as I don't like to judge, I do feel it leaves a very damaging impression, and having any relationship with them would be a challenge. I don't give them my time, and neither should you. You are not missing out on anything with such people. Just let go of it and don't let it fester in your mind, or you will start to have resentment and feel bad about yourself. Don't make the meaning of it about you. Again, notice how children can let go so easily, and how resilient they are. I love children so much.

It is not worthwhile; those so-called people pleasers, who overpromise and under deliver, have harmed themselves more than you ever could, so let go and stop trying to change them. You can only change yourself, and letting go without judgement of them, with peace and forgiveness, is something we must all work on. It's that peace that paves the way to delivering good health too.

Sometimes you can't help but come across them as they seem to be in your circle. For me, it's in business, and when I do come across them, I am polite to them, because I don't burn my bridges—but my time and how I engage is controlled and managed. Sometimes they have a big ego and think too much of themselves, and I feel that energy straight away. It is really quite strong, so I walk the other way before they start to penetrate my good energy fields and suck it out.

I just wish they would wake up and get some help dealing with the reasons behind such ways; but alas, without awareness and introspection, how can they? Their big egos will not let them.

We are born to be happy and to make people happy, so go ahead and do just that, and receive that thing that seeks to please you with an open heart. Being grateful and generous are values that can really help you here.

Question for you:
"In what way can you truly love yourself more?"

Guiding principle:
"Giving unconditional love is a way of receiving unconditional love."

Chapter principle:
"Healthy children are the closest to their own intuitive power.
They instinctively know how to balance themselves.
We come along and teach them to give up this power,
leaving them with a contaminated adult mind. If that's you,
reconnect back to your inner child, and lead from your intuitive
power about how you need to balance your health."

Chapter 8
Consistency Is Your Brand

How Key Is Consistency?

I can't stress enough the importance of consistency; without it, there is slow progress toward anything. There are more opportunities to self-sabotage because of inconsistent outcomes and results, and before you know it, you have taken many steps backwards. To then take steps toward your goals and dreams, it will take much more effort, and longer. One thing about consistency is that if your life and health is where it is, and not where you want it to be, then most likely your thoughts and actions are not aligned to what you want, so there is no real force behind keeping consistent.

When it comes to health, you need razor sharp focus, the kind of focus that business entrepreneurs talk about for success in business and financial goals. Some of these interventions include and suggest being consistent with your thinking and your actions, and doing what works and is getting the results that you desire. This means consistent evaluation of the strategy and its outcomes so that it propels you toward it with a certain pace, urgency, and commitment, and you get a taste for the outcomes, which will help you even during trying times. In health, the same principles apply but are more difficult to implement for some people, and so many give up easily because the changes are not tangible enough. Health for all is about a state of being, as well as having an optimally functioning physical body and mind. But how do we measure that like we measure net worth or profits in business? Furthermore, there are not many that have this because we don't focus on that.

So what remains is that our measure of health is the lack of illness or being fit, having the correct weight, being thin, having good skin and hair. This is fine at a point in time, but health is on a spectrum and is ever-changing and moving from one place on the spectrum to another, and as long as you can really truthfully look at your lifestyle as well, we cannot really know what is going on inside our bodies; and those changes, good and bad, take time to show up. I know plenty of people who have a combination of those attributes I mentioned earlier, yet their diet and level of stress are absolutely terrible. They count themselves really lucky, but without wanting to annoy them, physiological changes are going on deep inside, so it is only a matter of time before something detrimental shows up. The worrying trend, as always, is how young people don't look after their health anymore, and when they are a little older, that's the worst time to have to deal with it. We have to start from day one and continue to build on healthy foundations right into old age. This way, you will live longer and be well throughout your life, and be able to do whatever you want, like travel the world. If your health is really good today, and it is where you want it to be, then that would be the result of the attention you gave it in the past. If it's not, then again, that is what you did and did not pay attention to in the past; you can learn from that and action it from now on.

Make that your aim, and you will find momentum to keep going. If you are parents or want to be, I urge you to think about healthy living for you and your children, from the onset. You will give your children great foundations to take into adulthood. They will be special and on a different trajectory than other children are on in their health outcomes today. You will know and find the momentum to keep going. Have patience. The journey to health is probably the most unique experience you can ever have—it's a state of being, and you will notice it through subtle changes. You need to learn how to connect to your body in order to know it and trust it. It is speaking to you at every given moment. For health to be felt and seen continuously, you need to know that it's okay on the inside, and that it is in a confident state— that all your mechanisms, organs, and cellular transactions are at their optimum or working toward optimal wellbeing. Your body can also be a mechanistic platform to hear what is being processed in your mind, as long as you are willing to hear the truth. Come up with something that works for you, and then do it consistently until you get the results you want. It's not enough that you have health; you have to keep wanting it, one step at a time but consistently.

It's important to just get started, without overthinking and then freezing. Health in everyone differs, and unless it is an emotional goal, it may be a little hit and miss when you first start. By all means, experiment and play around with getting your health blueprint, with the principles at its core from this book, but don't ever give up.

If you think about the area in which most miracles are asked for, it's in health. It is the only defining attribute that has the capacity to cripple you for life, so why are we taking our health and that of our loved ones, so much for granted. Does ill health have to break you down mentally, physically, and spiritually for you to take notice? What is it going to take? The number one thing, in order to feel and have total freedom, is to have good health.

It is only when we experience a significant impact from a detrimental lifestyle, that we actually start to think about what life is, what we want, and what is important to us.

You see those people who have been given a second chance to live, and what they do and how much attention they pay to their health, because they know that the preciousness of life depends on it, and how important it is to empower others to understand how precious life is, through their experience of almost dying before their time. They become evangelical about it as if they have found something in themselves that needed a voice—a powerful voice. Having health is about being alive, really alive. It is not to be ridiculed or laughed at. It is a true gift.

Do you really want to put your health against a lottery, or do you prefer to drive it forward and upwards, and take back some control, being fully responsible and accountable? You may not get a second chance at life if you realise things way too late. Statistics for people's health round the globe, and in particular, the developed Western countries, are not on your side. Don't justify ignoring your health and the priority it deserves, by having thoughts like, "When I have time," or "There's too much going on, and I can't focus on it," or " I am okay; I only live once, so I might as well have a party every day." You deserve better than that, and your loved ones deserve better from you. It is about priority and discipline. Consistency becomes your ally in your road map to better health, with no interference from anything or anyone. Consistency is decisions in motion. It is also a transferrable skill that once you know how to use it with health, you will have this key internal resource in other areas of life. If you are getting results because of consistency in something, then using this same principle will help you in your health goals. The beauty of this is that you already have an internal resource equipped to help you in your health too, or in any other area of importance that is not quite firing on all cylinders.

Make sure your consistent ways with health are beneficial and progressive, and that the aspect of balance comes into play here too. I see many at each end of the health spectrum: those who really don't give a damn about their health or anyone else's, and those that are obsessed—neither is ideal. I have met some people who live, breathe, and conduct every aspect of health to perfection, but looking underneath as I like doing, it is more about control. It's their crutch, and it is not pleasant being around them. There is a difference between obsession about health and focus. Keep it in perspective— somewhere in the middle would be good—so that you can be consistent with it but relaxed at the same time.

Consistent wellness is the foundational life blood of positive and life enhancing results for you.

Most people tend to find it easier to consistently action bad habits like drinking, smoking, overworking, and overeating, and yet find it difficult to consistently go for a swim or eat healthy each day. That should be telling you that what you focus on is what you get, and that there is an inner conflict that exists between what you wish for and what you can't help in yourself. So whatever bad habits you have for your overall health, think about how consistently you entertain those habits, and how definitive the outcome is for you—but at least you know about consistency. Now imagine if you could create better habits that are more in tune with your future health and wellbeing. What are they, and what do you need in order to put them in place to achieve that?

Question for you:
"What habits are you repeating like a pro?"

Guiding principle:
"No change to better health is going to happen
unless you really really want it."

The Value of Consistency

Focusing on what you want to achieve is what consistency needs to be building. These actions allow for focus, clarity, and motivation toward the end goal, an aspect that works toward whole health. We are all accustomed to doing things that are meaningful once or twice, and yet expect sustainable results. It is not ever going to happen; it is a sheer fluke, which you cannot repeat or duplicate.

Consistency is a trait or methodology that gives duplicity. We are badly trained in the illusion that people who have what you want were just lucky, but if you were to look into their ways, they were constantly taking action, which gave them the amazing results, like wealth, investment portfolios, property portfolios, success and millions in business, and happy harmonious relationships. It is wonderful that some of them want to share their wealth of wisdom and experience, and take to the stage to speak and empower the rest of us so that we can learn and hopefully implement some of their teachings—after all, it is our duty to share things that transform lives for people who are ready.

Let's have a look again at this, in the health aspect. When is going to the gym once or twice or on an adhoc basis, going to achieve fitness and agility? When is eating healthily every now and again, going to change your eating for benefit? Would Olympic champions achieve their medal status by training only when they felt like it? They have to push themselves every day for that kind of success, be fed by their ambition, intuition, and motivation, and be guided by feedback from their coaches and their own physical and mental intellect. What you want, and the magnitude of your ambition and goal, will dictate what you have to do and when.

The results and outcomes are always a consequence of what you focus on, and if you focus on it consistently over a period of time, the results will come faster.

In today's world, doing something consistently that you are not used to is a real problem. We get influenced easily, and we can steer off path. There is a reason that top athletes hire coaches: It is their job to impress consistency, and to keep their athletes accountable to the behaviours that will get the results they desire. But even a coach is not present 24/7, so they still have to manage themselves correctly. Good coaches empower their coachees to coach themselves during these times. They may not be physically training, but they have to be just as strong mentally. It gives me so much pleasure to hear myself in others, even after years have gone by. It may be a phrase or an empowering word that surfaced during our coaching interface, and they know what made the difference, and they hold onto it as a precious gemstone of increasing value. It was a moment or a particular session that turned it round for them—it's quite remarkable. You have to be coachable, but not everyone is, even if they think of themselves as open-minded at any given time. Coaching is more than just having a conversation or being a good listener; it's being skilled, and the bigger skill is doing it naturally and in harmony, not as an extension of you but as a part of you, and the moment of impact is what they remember and absorb, so that they can use that insight to coach themselves as well, and into their future years.

Many will accept coaching because they are stuck somewhere, but as soon as they find a solution to it, they go off; and sometimes they cannot sustain themselves in this new way. So, only bring yourself to coaching if you are up for the ride—a much deeper ride. If I had it my way in the world, everyone would get a coach, because it is just as important to have that holding space during good times too. Coaching each other can become a truly genuine community enterprise. Imagine our children having a coach right by their side—someone and something consistent in their life, evolving side by side as life evolves. I daresay that we would all have a consistent and most wonderful experience in life. I am not saying that this means there will not be challenges and problems in your life, but learning to deal with them in a healthy balanced way has to be a good thing. I use the term "evolve" as opposed to "thrive," because there is learning in it, and we can learn from the good stuff as well as the bad.

So how do we get consistent action for something we desire? It comes down to a few elements: planning and deciding on what it is you want, being specific and very clear as to what it looks and feels like, connecting to it as if you are already there, living it, having it, really firing up your motivation and desire for it, keeping it long term, listening and being aware of feedback, and not allowing yourself to get off track.

The way the skill of consistency works is by giving you the means to achieve whatever that it. It is one of the success principles. To achieve and have health by your side every day, consistency with good health practices will be the only way you will get it, maintain it, and keep it for life. Remember, I am not talking about any acute illness that comes around from time to time from a cold or virus, or an accident, but with health on your side, you will regain yourself easily and restoratively, and quickly, and there are rarely any complications.

To be honest, consistency with health was the hardest thing that I ever came across, and it took me years to figure it out. The usual excuses were children and money and time, and so many others, and when I ignored it long enough, I fell ill with diabetes. It took all my strength to reverse it; I did not want that to be a part of my life, and despite having a very hectic and active career and family life, I started to get insight about me as an evolving person, and about my ways and principles and values I held dearly, and the principles in this book were given birth. They all helped me so much, and to this day, still do. They helped my clients and also my children, and particularly helped me to have boundaries in place, further being consistent with exercise, eating, and sleeping well—all these things we take for granted because something more urgent comes about that we need to deal with.

It is true that the majority of people who fall off the wagon prioritise something else, like finances or too great a social life, and they say that the timing is wrong, and that their children are the priority. These are all rated far, far higher than one's health and wellness, and even if they had started, it would be the first thing that would be ditched, to be taken up later when convenient.

Consistency helps embed a habit, and as long as the habit is for health and wellness, it is a practice that is needed in order to make it easier and a part of your daily fabric.

The problem with ditching health and wellness for yourself, under this illusion that you can't do it at the same time as something else, is that you eventually start to feel guilty and bad about yourself, and that you let yourself down, and sacrificed yourself for this and that; so that does not work long term, and opens up the creation of other problems. How about protecting yourself from ditching your health, regardless of how the circumstances around you change? Don't make health and wellness so rigid that it can't adapt to change. Your health has to be in harmony with your life and desires, and paid the rightful attention it deserves. The skill is doing it all at the same time.

When you are in your best health, you will know; it is a state of being, and the energy within you and around you is quite extraordinary. You just know. It's a feeling that far surpasses normal, and you start seeing things shifting for the better in every way—that's when it gets to be real fun and a life lived.

Many people, when it comes to their health, are a bit too much dilly-dally. There are those who on one hand want their health but are not willing to come away from bad ways; and there are those who are just ignorant of it because they have no obvious and recognisable health challenges. There is a real lack of discipline in their ways with good health, which can also give them an insight into other areas of their lives.

Their boundaries can be too flimsy and easily broken or pushed in. They live from a free state, like that of a child, and life for them can be chaotic but somewhat spontaneous.

I look at the millions put toward cancer charities for research on a cure. Not all cancers are the same, and so the interventions have to be different, so why are we giving money to generic cancer charity companies—today's big businesses? Does it make it any sweeter that they are trying to find a cure by highlighting and penetrating your emotional bank to raise funds? We know that the risk of cancer increases if you are obese and lead a life of stress and anxiety, eat processed foods, and if your nutrition is depleted of whole foods and greens. It infuriates me that the drinking and eating culture in the UK is known worldwide, encouraging each other to go out of their minds by drinking gallons of beer and eating the dirtiest of foods, and then trying to raise money for cancer, by going on a sponsored walk, in remembrance of a loved one that has died of cancer. This is a disconnected way of living and truth. Another conflict is when cancer charities raise funds through cakes and coffee events, when they themselves know that sugar creates an unhealthy foundation to health. So what is really happening here? Are they so far removed from the history of the point that started the charity in the first place? No doubt that was a consequence for someone's personal pain. Is that not what most charities are rooted in?

I am not proud to belong to a human race that is intent on destroying each other and our planet.

What I do, when I help people (as do so many of my colleagues in the health sector) with their health, is hard, and what I write in this book is written from my heart, because that money that is given to charities like this, can be instead given to so many vulnerable in our world. We can build schools and educational facilities, and build a better and fairer healthcare system for everyone. We can work together to redistribute wealth so that we all have a good chance for health in our lives. Such charities have powerful marketing facilities, and these messages can pass by all logic in our brains, and gain an emotional charge so that we act with our money. Think about it: Why do charities get adverts on television during Christmas? Because they know that this is the time of year that the human spirit is more giving and more loving to each other than any other time. There has to be a fundamental shift in health for each of us to be accountable to ourselves and each other, or this type of illusion will go from strength to strength. Why is it that there are so many people that have cured their cancer, and needed no help from these charities? What did they do to get it back to where it should be? Most will say that they woke up and consistently took better care of themselves, and still do. They are alive, with renewed vigour! I know there are different cancers that need medical intervention and more research, but it begs the question of where our money is going and to who. The point is the hypocrisy, and just because they are a fuzzy-feeling charity, it gives them the mask to really just be running a business that is keeping us sick, feeding us lies, and playing on our emotions and their vulnerabilities with the media's portrayal of how bad cancer is. It is equal in devastation as any other illness, like diabetes. Let's start by saying no to fundraising with coffee and cake. If you have been to one of these, there is always 3x more cake than coffee, with people nicely chomping on excess sugar, under the illusion that they are doing a good thing. I did once, and a few months later saw adverts about sugar and obesity and cancer all being connected, and that was when I woke up to it. I hope you do too.

So, make a decision with your health and the health of the world—it really does start with you. Set an intention now! That's what kicked my diabetes into touch many years ago. No doctor or nurse could ever encourage that in me. I had to do that for myself. Well, let me tell you that healthcare is changing, and the patient's voice is louder than ever before—it needs to be recognised as real evidence, not tampered-with evidence.

Question for you:
"What is your relationship with consistency in anything,
and then with anything related to your health?"

Guiding principle:
"To achieve health for everyone,
you have to do your bit in the whole puzzle."

See It from the Other Person's View

Consistency in something is your brand, so to speak, because it is what you do to get results. It's not so important how you do it but the fact that you are doing it. It's not about a race or quick results, but it is a way to sustainable and longer-term outcomes. Through the journey, what is actually going on is a level of mastery. Consistency gives you mastery because it is your decision and intention in motion, and when you do it, it paves the way to learning more about yourself in a progressive forward-facing way.

Like I said earlier, it's one of your success principles.

Most people know someone who is on and off diets, but if you look at the overall progress, they are either fatter or the same. Is that because diets don't work? No, it is not, and it is in fact evident that many people in the industry make loads of money claiming this illusion that diets don't work. Most who head up weight loss have never been fat themselves or understand it enough to really help their customers, but they have to slate one thing in order to create noise for their solution, whether that is good or bad. What gets people hooked on their programmes is clever marketing and the courage to step up and claim a share of the market. We see social media entrepreneurs today like no other time, because it is so easy for people to believe in new solutions. There is never only one solution for getting ill health, whatever that looks like, to good health. Gaining and losing weight, and the ensuing obesity crisis, cannot be fixed only by eating well and counting calories or exercising more. There is a systematic change from education, personal health ownership, and the whole pipeline of food, both fresh produced and processed stuff, that has to be challenged. That is a big deal! And it is going to take every single one of us, one person at a time, to change it; and the best way is to prevent it in the first place.

Now, the problem that people have with sticking to anything that gets them to better health, is them themselves. It is the people that do diets that need to work on themselves. They get in their own way. We all have the potential to take on anything and MAKE it work if we really want to, and that comes from within.

When diets don't work, what is being dismissed or discounted is that the person did not allow for the diet to work—they could not or did not stick to the structure of it—in other words, they self-sabotaged themselves. They were not ready for the change, and they thought that they could do it their way and still get the same results; and above all, they could not provide consistency. People think that they have to have a constant environment in order for anything to be easy. Well, you have heard, I am sure, that everything worthwhile is not always easy.

No, YOU provide consistency, and YOU are the constant—it is what you choose—it is an internal resource that you provide by having a thought-through, self-supported attitude. As far as I am concerned, all diets work; anything can work—it just depends on YOU.

It is intriguing that people who have never been fat say that diets don't work. I would not go to anyone that presents weight loss in their solutions for people, when they themselves have never been fat. It makes absolutely no sense whatsoever, as it's more about textbook theory and teachings rather than real life solutions. It is only the experience in you that brings the greatest value. In the same way, good health is not about textbook theory or tons of clinical studies and papers; it's about experience and action.

You can't give to others what you have not had yourself.

It is important to get support for people around you, and that may not happen if you cannot commit to what you want for yourself in health. You could be on and off diets, or decide that you want to start running, and train yourself for that; whatever it is, if you don't commit and stick to it, what will their perception be of you? Have you asked? Do they challenge you or support you to keep going, or do they feel sorry for you and encourage you to give in?

It is quite normal for people watching you by your side to become skeptical of whether you will ever get it done. Can you blame their skepticism?

So, here is the thing: Consistency in your habits, aligned with your health goal or any other goal in life, is aligned to getting you faster results. It builds your brand, and people can begin to trust you to do what you say you are going to do. That, in health, is very important. The support, when it's trusting and trusted, is critical.

I have been there many times, not sticking to things I had carefully planned out and knew were proven to work. I lacked consistency with it, finding ways round things, and being all into it one day and all out another day. I broke my own set boundaries, and allowed other views to infiltrate my better judgement and my health goals for my body and mind. I was confused and did not see consistent results, and that meant throwing in the towel and giving up. There were also plenty of opportunities for feedback from loved ones I lived with, and they knew what I was like and my triggers, better than I did for myself, yet it was so frustrating to hear them tell me. They knew my blind side, and had I listened, there were many chances to get things back on track. So you can imagine what others have to also go through, and it is understandable that they can also lose sight of what you can and can't do. It is like calling a bluff. They don't know if you are being serious or if it's just another thing you are going to try having a go at.

The hardest thing for me was to lose weight after pregnancy. Even going from a first-time diabetic to a non-diabetic was easier than losing the excess weight I had put on, but when the goal became part of something bigger and more urgent, I found a structure for myself and stuck to it consistently until I got the results I wanted. In fact, I got more than what I had planned, which was a great bonus. I went from a size 24 to a small 16—that was 4 dress sizes down, in less than 5 months; and although I had always hovered between sizes 10/12, my size 16 was good enough, and I felt happy and have maintained that till now. I would now like to take it back down and achieve a healthy size 12/14.

So, you see, if you declare something to someone and then don't do it, it speaks very loudly about you. Is that a judgement? Yes, partly, but we come back to the meaning of trust and influence. People need to believe that what you say, you can do for yourself, or that you have found a way around your own challenges, or are at least working toward it with some level of success. It's not about perfection or not showing your vulnerabilities or setbacks. The journey has the better value to inspire and motivate, even if not the finished article. The sad fact is that the declaration or disclosure publicly means that you have to take it seriously. How many people, who are changing their health for the better for themselves, are open and honest about it because of rejection, judgement, or fear of failure? Not many. That's actually because it is more to do with what we think of ourselves and the fact that we can't stick to things consistently, that we don't trust ourselves.

Imagine that you can trust yourself.

To get anywhere near the result we want, we need to declare exactly what we want, and then go about setting ourselves goals to achieve it no matter what. A timeframe is helpful because it gets you focused, and if you are competitive like me, then a time frame and something that is a challenge is great.

So declare to your world the way you want to live—your health goals, your financial goals, and so on—and don't be afraid. Get into a consistent pattern of whatever you need to do that will bring the desired outcome to you; and by the way, it should not end there, because in health, for example, that's something we all need for the rest of our lives—it is a progressive and forward journey. It has the capacity to raise us all higher than we ever imagined, and it needs to start from day 1; and if not then, whatever age you are, start now—not tomorrow—NOW!

What you say, is your brand; and it engages some very important values, which are integrity and reliability. It is very important for me to do what I say I will do, and if for whatever reason I just can't, then I hold my hand up and say that too, but I work on adapting it so that I can still reach my goals, even if it takes a little longer.

Remind yourself what you want the outcome to be.

So this brings us back to what you want in your life. From a health perspective and through choices, remind yourself what you had put down at the beginning chapters of this book, and do an audit to check if those items are still true or if they need changing, deleting, or adding to.

A very powerful way to engage both parts of your brain is to do a vision board depicting everything you dream about, through all channels of life: money, health, family, social, travel and adventure, fun, and so on. Get as creative as you can, and do it from your heart—make sure it's fully yours and not what your parents want for you, if different! When done, by all means upload your completed vision boards, and tag #visionboardforhealth. Please visit www.SanjayaPandit.com

My vision for people living the life of their dreams starts with looking after themselves. There is enough advice on business and commerce, how to grow rich, and how to develop interpersonal skills, and all this is fantastic information for us all, but there is not enough for being healthy from the beginning. Even entrepreneurs need to take note. I have met and seen many who are brilliant at what they do, and I have seen how successful they are, what they can inspire in us and teach us, and how some can motivate us, but there is something lacking in many: their health. They have achieved great success at the expense of their health, even though that was never an intention. Too much of today's crisis in health has been left to sort out by someone else, even divine grace; and as much as I believe in God, I think we are equipped with tools to help ourselves—at least, let us all respect that. I have beliefs and faith, but I also take full responsibility for my stuff, and I know that we don't have to sacrifice our health while chasing our other dreams. We can achieve health with other achievements; it is simply a matter of knowing how to do it.

The information currently available is a bit all over the place. Health affects every one of us, and anything living has to conceptualise health. Nature has a way of showing good health and ill health, and it's when we are not listening or paying attention that we get ourselves into a mess. This book gives you basic principles encompassing and framing three key areas of our wholeness. Within this, there is room for people to integrate their knowledge, seek other knowledge, and have opportunities to work things out for themselves, and as long as they keep the three in balance, they can create a way that is ideal to them. How many people will say that to you? It's always about following someone else's way, from one year to another; and like I said, you are left feeling confused and out of sync. I would like very much to again acknowledge that one thing in health does fit all, and I choose to take a view above it all, higher up, as if I were in a helicopter, hovering and looking at my life below. From this place, I can see the outcomes people are looking for in their health. Some are ready, some are nearing a point of no return (even though I cannot imagine that even they cannot do something), and some don't know anything, and they frankly don't care; but they will also be ready like you someday soon, and then we can be ready to help them. My hope is for everyone to make a start or to continue the good work they are already doing.

So, remind yourself again and again what you want, and have it in a way that it is written or in pictures so that it acts as a structural reminder, every given moment, of whether you are on course or not. Of course, there needs to be some wiggle room and flexibility, and sometimes we will have to get off path to realise the value of getting back on it, or change our path for even greater things.

If you don't know what you want, then go back to the beginning, and get yourself a pen and paper and read through each point; reflect on it before you move on to the next point. This is written in a format that helps to build you up. It builds up momentum and passion for an exciting, healthy possibility of life, by bringing you awareness. Read the book as many times as you want; the penny will drop at the right time, when your mind is fully open to the information and insight. Answer the questions I ask of you throughout the book.

A vision around health in your life, and in that of your family and children, needs to be specific, and points made in this book can be used so that you are fully integrating health in all its facets, because some areas will have more meaning and priority for people than others; but it does need to be named, discussed, talked about, and consistently weaved into your daily living. It is like the base and foundation that make-up artists use, without which the finish on top cannot be flawless and seamless.

So, connect your vision with what is important to you and what you want this life to look and feel like. Engage all sensory mechanisms to this vision for yourself, like smell, sight, touch, sound, and intuition. Start using such mechanisms to access your intuition and dreams, with a quiet mind and state. Imagine access to your most powerful brain, your subconscious mind, which is where patterns are based to drive our behaviours.

Limiting paradigms and beliefs can be based here, and it's a hell of a driver—you need access to it in order to change it or to put other forms of deliberate thinking in its place.

Just like a quick snap of your fingers, you can start again, and if I can and did, ANYONE CAN and will. We can only survive if we can access what is given to us from nature, our spiritual kingdom, and each one of us is given a gift to pass on and share with the world. Imagine what the possibilities could then be. When you get optimal health, it's like a rebirth—a second chance. It's only when you feel genuinely clean and well that you don't know how unwell you actually felt. Many people try to swim in the darkest drudge—it is heavy and burdensome, and it's hard to breathe with their health crisis. I don't want my life to end because of ill health or that I brought death to myself before it was time. I want to have lived in every way possible—to my inherent potential—and for the reason for my birth, my body serving me to live a higher life; and then when the time comes, as it will for all of us, I get to leave a legacy in my world, or even to the world, that can be passed on to many generations, present and future. It is only then that I would be able to truly rest in peace and free my spirit.

Question for you:
"How do others see you in the pursuit of good health?
How do you see yourself?"

Guiding principle:
get support from people in your quest for good health,
they have to trust you and you them. Have integrity."

Consistent Higher Standards and Expectations

The desire to be, think, and act differently and uniquely is not celebrated in most of our daily environments. Having higher expectations and standards that make you stand out can be lonely initially, and difficult in most cases, but for health, this is also an aspect that is proving to be important, changing health for the better, not just for you but for everyone around you. Despite the temporary downside of discomfort, it is essential if we are going to make an impact on the world, for all of us to enjoy better health and not endure illness for longer than we need to. And so having higher standards for self-health firstly, is golden. From there, the ripple effect will be felt in others more than you could ever know.

Raising personal goals and standards, and belief in good health and all its benefits, is a gift to everyone, including you. I have worked in healthcare long enough to know how contradictory that can be for people. The standards of personal health are inconsistent and sometimes very poor. There are societal and financial inequalities that make self-health difficult, but I also see it as an excuse that people can hide behind. There are so many ways to start and then raise standards for yourself as you move along this journey. It doesn't matter in the end where you come from or what you are born into; health can only start for you when you intend it in the correct manner. Without your heart and mind engaged, it will never be, and any book or true health guidance won't make any difference.

It's like with anything; until you truly understand the benefits and are grateful for that—and in this case, for good health—you will dismiss the importance and value of it. You have to want it, and truly want it, like the air you breathe. And why wait for the end of your life to finally understand that?

During all my years in healthcare, and even now, I know that there is such a lack of respect for one's health. People have to literally be sick to want it back; and then, for many, despite being sick, they just continue to abuse their bodies, their minds, and their hearts and spirits. Why? Because they take it so much for granted. That lack of responsibility, gratitude, and ownership can bring devastation to their lives, and more importantly, to the people they leave behind.

Let's help ourselves and protect those we love by being fully around, by being alive in body, mind, and spirit.

That means raising your standards and expectations without becoming silly about it. I am not a fan of those who are at the extreme end of health. The problem with that is that it can be an assault on their mental health. I know this because I have worked with them, and also with the people that have to live with them. Anything that is so addictive in thoughts, behaviours, and actions—if not balanced—can be harmful in the long run, and actually shut you down. So, I like health without fads, and without evangelical living and the pushing of an aggressive sell. If you are having to push a certain way, or are having a certain route to health pushed down your throat, it may not be genuine and sincere long term, and the weight of the person or group pushing it is largely for their benefit, at your expense. You may ask, am I not pushing the same?

No, I am not. How can I be, because wanting you to have good health, and using these principles, is something that comes to you when you are born to live. The way that having health is promoted is piecemeal, and I want to bring the concept that you have to work on these various elements of yourself, at the same time, to have health and to maintain health. Those are within you. They are the foundations that people ignore, and without having those in place, they go about searching for something that is marketed and promoted—fads that give them a false hope in what they think they desire. Without having the foundations, it's going to be very shaky and cannot work long term. My view is that if you have these principles in place, and you work hard to develop them and maintain them, without going to the dark side as they say, you may not need anything else. If you get these principles into your children, and get them to understand them and maintain them, then we are going to have a healthier, brighter, and more energetic future for them and all future generations.

Raise your standards of care and expectations for the health of others, and voice your concerns to anyone who is not grounded in their health, and who you can clearly see is abusing that. Say it, name it, and be courageous. Sitting on the fence is an assault of your human duty to be the best and to bring out the best in everyone that crosses your path or stays in your life.

My concept of health is about raising those standards; you have a responsibility to yourself and to others that love you. This way, there is room for adaptation, uniqueness, and ingenuity from within. It is then positioned much higher up, directly linking to your best and higher self. It's a way of being conscious and mindful.

Believe me, you won't be a bore or even a social imposter, because when you are truly healthy, you are charismatic and soulful, and the rays of sunshine from you are brighter. Demand rightful change to your health and that of others. Raise your standards of healthcare, and expect higher standards for others—eating better and in smaller portions, eating good quality food, having good movement and exercise—it can be introspection with gratitude and appreciation. It is about being in union with your higher self, carefully redeeming the thoughts that keep you from breathing, and remembering to be grateful each day for your blessings. Let's have faith and commitment in humanity, and show kindness always to ourselves and others. Bring the best version of yourself to your world and to the greater world, and always be in awe of all life and our wonderful planet Mother Earth.

Do this as if you mean business, and do it consistently so that it becomes you, and you, it. If you see that in someone else, open them to it. The easier it feels to understand and appreciate such people, the more evidence it is that you are moving up to your higher self with love. There is a lot of good in our world, and there is more of it than not. We have learnt to not recognise it, to devalue it, and to be weary of it.

Question for you:
"What standards and expectations can you raise for yourself
when it comes to your health?"

Guiding principle:
"It does not matter where you are, who you are,
or where you have been; there is always a choice of seeing
and doing good through your health."

Chapter principle:
"Without consistency, action thoughts,
and behaviours, you will not achieve what you want.
Make your determination for good health a must,
and commit to it. It's your choice and fully in your power."

Integrating Health into Everyday Life – The Gift, the Vision, and the Legacy

Chapter 9
Your Gift

Your Parenting Style

I want health to be an important aspect of your life from day one, in an ideal world, which means starting at the beginning. Much of my book covers aspects of health that are simply too important and vital for overall mental, physical, emotional, and spiritual health to be good and sustainable for life. It has to be not just talked about holistically but practiced that way, and not by seeing 10 different practitioners and health care professionals, but by putting you in charge of yourself and thus impacting others in a positive way—what we can do with our duty and opportunity to change the lives of thousands of children, and children of the future, so that their experience of life is far more enhanced, yet simplified.

Now, if you are not a parent and have some way to go, but you have come to this point in the book, I want to invite you to continue reading the final chapters. Remember that I mentioned that there is a childlike part of you, as well as a parent part of you. These are ego states, as I said, but they are important parts of you that do need some attention as they drive your communication and thought patterns, depending on communication and what ego state is operational. So, imagine that you are in your childlike ego state—what do you notice about yourself that is childlike, in your tone, gestures, behaviours, thoughts, and beliefs? I ask the same question of you when you are in your parent ego state: Can you hear or see in your mind, anyone specific, like your mum or dad or grandad or aunt? Who are you most like when you are here? And again, this depends on the functionality of this parent-ego state; it could be challenging you or criticising you, or lovingly nurturing you and encouraging you to be your best, or it may want you to be so free that nothing has any boundaries, and you live a life without boundaries.

Please think and gain some awareness of this before you read on, as it will make more sense in your parenting style with your kids and, of course, yourself.

If you are a parent, you will know firsthand how parenting is an incredible mix of skills. Please give gratitude to your parents or a similar role model that helped raise you, whatever you think of them; and I hope it is with love, and that you can appreciate all their efforts. It is a hard job, and not everyone is proficient at it; they have to learn as they go along. It is a skill; practicing and trusting yourself makes it a lot easier.

How we parent largely depends on our experiences and parenting styles that we witnessed when we were children. I still believe that we can choose how we parent, despite our experiences, and we have to be able to adapt our parenting style today. These next principles are about nurturing, self- care, and giving the correct attention and recognition to that part of you, from the parent to the child, whether literally or via your ego states, which again are communication patterns set up in the three parts of yourself that give you your personality. This is the work of Eric Berne via transactional analysis, whereas ego is from Sigmund Freud's theory on id, ego, and super-ego.

Let me first get the irony and mismatch out of the way when it comes to messages from parents: It is important to understand that even if you say nothing, your actions and gestures are still doing the talking! Some examples of this mismatch between how parents are with their children, and how they are with themselves, causes a mismatch, and some can be of concern. So, for example, I have worked with mums who would be very careful of what they gave their kids to eat, but were somewhat lax with their own food, giving in to their childlike ego state that wanted sweets and treats, which they would not allow their own kids to have. Then I have worked with dads who were very present and compassionate with their kids' misgivings and, at times, failures, but were highly critical of themselves and about the smallest, most insignificant things. And then there were those who were very loving to themselves but could not show that kind of love to their kids, and expected way too much from them.

These mismatches are very interesting, and when it was pointed out to them, it also was a surprise to them, and new knowledge and learning would help them change their ways.

Parenting, today, is a whole lot more challenging because today's children are so quick and learn things way before their time. We have less peer support and knowledge about parenting that is structured around our family values, because families are living apart from each other. Every new couple is encouraged to live in their own married home so that they can be independent and lead a largely private life. There is nothing wrong with that, but there is also value in those families that can stay together somehow, or have a close bond where there is much communication between them, in a deeper way rather than just arbitrary banter such as who's going to be with who, during important traditional celebrations.

Whatever your ways, and whatever you teach, the power of influence, as parents to your young ones, is greater than you may think. It is a very important and significant role, and one that can vary from culture to culture. There is no one way of parenting, and no perfect way. There are many variables—it is the most diverse and dynamic area of life. I personally like mixing things up, taking the best from my own culture and from other cultures, heritage, and our modern culture, but it has to be congruent with my own values, and add a welcome and open depth to my parenting style and to their experience as a little and young human being. Some cultures insist on certain methods, and if they don't resonate, I don't take it on board. My goal for my children, as always, has been one where they are not just my children but children of a much happier, bigger world, so they can contribute meaningfully to the sustainability of mankind and the planet, and so that they can have an international presence and become truly aware and integrated global citizens. There are certain things that we can create and make constant in parenting across any culture and traditions, which preserves the longevity of that little person we have just brought into this world.

With health having its deserved place in cultures and the coaching of health, with every child and that part in you, can you imagine them being taught skills such as coaching, communication, and mindfulness, right from the beginning of their precious lives? What mainstream school or education facility teaches that? None! It has so much mileage as far as setting an intention and agenda that is so clear for their health, that that becomes the cornerstones for life together. In this process, parents, men and women, can also be better, live better, and do better. Without a multidimensional change process, we will get more of what we have today: everyone grappling with disjointed health and wellbeing, from a place of illness or its fearful avoidance. Let's develop proactive insight and an attitude for good health for everyone.

I am blessed with four children, and I have practically raised them by myself, teaching them as much as I know, and making sure that when I learn something new and value it, it will also benefit them in their life, so I share it and explain it, without shoving it down their throats as some evangelical behaviour.

I am sure you know that children and teenagers are notorious for not always engaging, but don't stop giving out wisdom and teaching them despite feeling like you are talking to a brick wall, because it does catch on, and when they are ready to pay it attention, they will; and they will use it or repurpose it in ways that are far more creative than you could have first imagined. It is worthwhile; invest in the time to teach them good things: things that are not taught in school; things that will help them live a good healthy life, upskilling them in resilience, emotional intelligence, mindset, kindness, love for themselves, and confidence; and the role of compassion in their lives, and also their academic goals and desires at the same time.

There is still, in my view, plenty of outdated teaching through outdated beliefs and traditions that are harder to uphold, in which young people may not be interested. They live a life with so much diversity that it is hard to keep them, and us for that matter, on the straight and narrow; and like I said, I have raised my children to become global citizens, which means that I hope they are open to all sorts of experiences, people, and places, as well as different faiths and religions and worldly education.

Otherwise, what happens to people, like so many I know, is that they find it difficult to adapt to the "new," which causes them anxiety because they are so attached to protecting traditions and the culture from fading away. I am all for sharing the incredible wisdom that comes from my culture; in truth, it is truly fascinating and has such a great place in today's world, and my hope is that joining the forces of good from others will make the future world a much better place to live in with a larger group of people.

As with anything, there is a darker side, and it saddens me to see that people are so disconnected from their ways. This example is, luckily, in the minority, but why should it have a place in society at all? Some people pretend to be gracious, even religious for that matter; yet in their workplaces and businesses, they treat their staff with the lowest dignity, bullying them, controlling them, and eroding anything they may have left as a human being. I see that so much in my culture. I am sure this is everywhere. Our upside-down world makes it okay to dish out punishment for speaking up for yourself in class, but there is no punishment to those students who are bullies, who throw eggs at passing cars after their school day, whilst the whole group of youth laugh out loud, still wearing their school's uniform. When reports are made to the school, nothing gets done. Are schools so desperate for numbers and funding that they keep these students in? These same people will be adults one day, and one of our children will be working alongside them. Can you imagine being in the company of someone that was never sanctioned properly and feels that they can get away with it all their life? Who is responsible for these types of people? By tolerating such behaviours, we create potential monsters.

We are all responsible—the school, parents, police, and the person whose car was hit with eggs. We are all scared of disruptive youth, and more so when they collude in numbers these days. We don't speak up and give them clarity into what cannot be tolerated; instead, for a quiet, peaceful, and perceived safe life, we just try to ignore it and get on with our lives. How will that help anyone in the long-term?

Parenting skills today are about the balancing of time, giving and receiving information, teaching, learning on the go, and inspiring to get the best out of you and your children, and it shows one fundamental thing: your leadership style. Forget that you are a CEO of some massive corporation and are applauded for your leadership role in the company—is your home life falling apart? Your corporate leadership style doesn't work at home with people who are personal to you. Personally, leadership that has positive health outcomes for everyone, has to be developed at home, because it would be very different to the types of leadership in today's world. Imagine someone becoming a CEO of a company, who handles leadership with love and heart, and what potential that company would have to grow its people and its processes. We all need more of that profile in important roles, and not just to conquer and divide, which can be very masculine energy. The problem is that many don't think a softer approach to leadership is good enough, and that it is weak to lead with your heart. What will be weak and make you disconnect from yourself and all the people you lead, will be the same bullying, autocratic, one-dimensional male or female (that wear men's trousers) approach of today. This is the dilemma between aspiration of tomorrow and reality of today.

Leadership has to be multidimensional, all-inclusive, and engaging. We go to work under an illusion that we have no choice, that we have to sacrifice being dumped on every day by incompetence, and that we can ignore the disharmony for the sake of keeping our head above water—to do what? Pay someone else through bills, never quite managing to escape from financial commitments and insecurities, and each time, each day, your physical health, your mental health, your emotional health, and your spiritual health erodes, one piece at a time? When you finally get home and have some sort of anesthetic—wine, chocolate, or whatever—how can you parent from this place? You can't shut yourself in a room, even if that's all you want to do, because your kids depend on you feeding them, doing homework with them, and getting them ready for tomorrow. How can you parent and maintain health and wellbeing for them, from this place? The challenge is so real for many—I know; I have been there lots of times. It only started to change when I decided to work for myself and with myself.

Most parents have a two-week holiday in the summer, which won't rebalance anything for anyone.

Leadership starts in the home, and as parents, that is what we teach our children to be—their own leaders and masters. We are our own masters, and we must learn to lead ourselves before we can lead anyone else.

Think about your leadership style. What works and what doesn't? What comes naturally to you, and what doesn't? Have you been told to be different than you are, in order to fit in and be liked?

There is still tremendous hope that everyone in our families can be healthy, and know health as it is meant to be. What do you communicate for and against it? Become really clear and aware of this.

Question for you:
"What is your default parenting style? Even if not a parent, how do you parent yourself? Is it with love, criticism, or over nurturing?"

Guiding principle:
"Leadership is not about your title role;
it is an opportunity for you to influence kindness,
health, and compassion to others, who look to you equally
and with care so that you can bring out the best in them."

Time Spent Doing and Being, in Balance

Time is one of our most valuable resources and the one thing that most people have a very bad relationship with. It's how they choose time with certain elements of their life. We take great care to teach children to cross roads safely, to avoid going toward fire or touching plugs with live electricity. We even put sharp objects away until they learn how to handle them. The same efforts should be put toward teaching them about their health and how their bodies work, encouraging them to open their minds on how sleep is so important and why, rather than barking orders, "Go to sleep, it's past your bed time!" Like everything, we all need an understanding of why and how we do things, what the benefits are, and very importantly, if we are all sticking to the boundaries we have created for ourselves in life.

There are many boundaries enforced by the outside world that you do not agree to either—some you do, some you don't, and some you just ignore if you can get away with it. Take the 30-mile-an- hour speed limit on city roads, for example, if you are in the UK anyway, or any speed limit in your country. Be honest; have you complied with it always? Do you understand why that came to be law? Under what circumstances do you comply with it, and when don't you? I know that it was never explained to me why this was the case, and there are also other things that are enforceable without really understanding why or what the benefits are. Without real understanding, it just becomes inconvenient and hard to motivate yourself to stick to it. It was only when I broke the limit and got caught on camera during my early driving years that I opted for a speed awareness course and not points on my license. This course gave me evidence of what happens when I go over 30 miles an hour on city roads, and if there was to be a collision, accident, or a run in with a pedestrian, what their chances of survival would be. At 30 and below, quite a bit, but I was going at 34 miles an hour, and when you start approaching that speed and above, an accident can be serious and perhaps even fatal. I have seen a collision at 40 miles an hour, where there were people around, with schools and children and cyclists, and it makes you rethink. It is a matter of life and death.

For health, it's the same analogy. Explain why it is good for us to keep health always and to prioritise it, and they will already have an understanding. There are some who just won't get it, like in the course. Despite these videos affecting me, there were some men and women, of all ages, who were caught a few times over the years. They were not getting the message. They had not killed anyone as of yet; but boy, were they taking risks! To pay attention to health and wellness, it has to be an informed choice.

Too many parents are worried that they will lose authority with their children if they don't tell them off abruptly rather than using a softer, more discussion approach—involving them, explaining, and including them in decisions—because they may be faced with a struggle of wills. That makes life harder for the parents. Actually, you will be pleasantly surprised at their attitude when they are involved from a young age. When you are teaching them to think and challenge in a balanced way, with fresh perspectives, it is a skill they will not learn in education today, and it is great practice for later years. It's worthwhile, as good foundations never get wasted, but it takes effort and consistency from all involved, which is why it is easier to bark orders to little people. It is a good insight again into your motivation and leadership as parents.

Whatever ways you teach your kids, the power of influence from parents to their young ones is greater than what you may think. It is a very important and significant role. It is hard, challenging, and mixed with emotion, and yet incredibly fulfilling, and probably the best thing you will ever do. There are many of you reading this book who are not yet parents, or may choose not to be or can't be, but this is still relevant to yourself and to children that you come across through social circles, work, and play—whatever it is, you have a parental and child ego state within you that you can practice with, and this communication has to be healthy in order for you to be healthy.

Think about how much time goes into meaningless activity, discussion, and spending time with people that have no meaning and are actually unsupportive. Perhaps it is time to renegotiate your valuable time. Perhaps it is time to do things that have fulfillment and are important and will impact not just you but generations to come. Teaching them about good use of time, and how to make time for health daily, will bring a considerable number of benefits.

One of the ways that it is done best is to first understand how to structure your time. You can start by simply writing down groups of tasks and actions you take daily, and allocate the amount of time to devote to this. Then write all the things you are aware of that are missing, which you would like to do as well but don't get the time to do because your day and night is perhaps packed full of mundane things. Allocate time to what you want to do and who you want to do it with, including the full version of yourself, and allocate thoughts of how much time you can devote to this instead, which will result in a better way of life for you and those directly and positively affected by this change.

Once this has been done for the first time, devote time to practicing the new habits, and then devote time also to evaluate it after continuously doing it for 3 consecutive months.

It is really important that you include all areas of your life: work, travel, people, money, health, social, and so on. Please visit my website at www.SanjayaPandit.com for a bonus template on this, as well as for more information on using a time structure model created by Eric Berne, whose teachings on transactional communication patterns are very insightful. I use them and they are very much part of my overall unique coaching offer. It has helped me to redesign how I spend time daily on more meaningful things.

Question for you:
"How are you planning for good, sustainable whole health?"

Guiding principle:
"Much of our time is spent doing things on autopilot;
instead, be conscious and mindful, and use the time given to you
to do and be better—interrupt yourself from stagnation."

Teach Them the Value of Health from Day 1

By now, I hope you agree that health is much more than being fit and eating right, and that your health teaching system within your family and sphere is best designed and shared from day one, which means that it needs to be in the fabric of all our daily lives. The biggest responsibility any parent or guardian has is the wellbeing of themselves and that of their children. It has to be shared in a family system as far and wide as we can get it to be. We have to spend a lifetime maintaining this, and the quicker we start, the better we will be at maintaining it effortlessly. Imagine what lives we could have if this was an inherent system integrated into our lives every day. Health is fundamental and cannot be negotiated if we want a better and more connected and integrated version of ourselves! And you can take it with you anywhere you go. It's like owning a home; you have to consistently maintain it, and that takes time, effort, attention, and dedication, and it's constant. By the time you are finished a part of the house, something else is ready for attention. Ignore it, and it becomes a problem area that can be costly to fix.

If you are a parent and are reading this book, or are someone who can influence any child, I have so much hope for you to have a fantastic, enriching life together with your children, and to give them the biggest gift life has to offer. The idea that I can teach my children on values, how to educate themselves on academics and life, how to be charitable and kind, and how to have good relationships and a successful life, through an open mind, amounts to nothing if I can't teach them about how to preserve and be well, and how crucial that is. It is always my centrepiece, but it's fragile and can be dislodged by life's big curve balls. But if they know health or never lose sight of it, even while these curve balls hit, they can get it back anytime they want, and it is never lost forever. Let's teach them to live life, and to be truly alive and empowered by having health and wellness central to their being. Imagine soaking up the energy of such a being.

My goals for my children have always been for them to be full of energy and free of medication, even pain killers, as well as to keep their mind, body, and spirit healthy, and to tell them to look for answers they question on, from inside them and not just from outside influences. We can reduce the amount of chronic illness we see today, and the only way to curb its growth, as statistics predict, is if we stand up to it, take our health back to basics, take full responsibility, and challenge what in our world keeps us ill and reliant on drugs, with an inauthentic, inconsistent, and sometimes unethical and broken health care system.

The way to start is to utilise and make space for all the principles in this book, as well as any other that you resonate with. I have made and will make available lots of bonus tools that will help in these areas, and I have some fantastic programmes that have been developed and proven for easy implementation.

We have multiple forums and knowledge on parenting, on how to get the baby through the initial stage of their life, and guidance from health practitioners who are checking on sleep and routine feeding, baby yoga, and all the basics. The instinct of parents is very much for preservation and protection, and it's understandable with so much oxytocin circulating in their bodies through touch and loving attachment, but this changes as parenting becomes a bit more complex, and they are trying to juggle way too much. Much of the care given at the beginning, starts to subside, and many mothers go back to work and struggle to find time; they focus on the various and ever-evolving areas of their lives, diluting time and energy to keep things ticking. But as children grow, the opportunity to teach, guide, and coach them is so unlimited that it actually excites me how incredible they can be—not by barking orders at them, and not by leading them through fear and control, but by being a positive role model and being self-aware yourself.

What I now know about myself just came too late. Some may argue that I had to make mistakes and be challenged to find myself, but I know that there were traits about me, when I was a young girl, which I lost in the middle part of my life, and which were so important for me to claim back because that is who I was born to be, and who I am once again becoming. Many parents, at one point or another, ask themselves where those little innocent, cuddly babies have gone.

Some relish in the experience with them to that point, and some cannot recognise their children at all—whatever your experience, we all get a chance to mentor, coach, and bring out the best in people every day.

Life is challenging and unnecessarily complicated, and we are not very good at holding up our hands and asking for help, or acknowledging or even surrendering to the fact that we are not being our best, and instead seek to change it. We have to have the desire to reclaim it, and become ever more aware and enlightened that we are not being the best we can be—and I want to change that.

Kids press our buttons at times when we don't expect it. When we are tired and our own tanks are empty, the last thing we need is our kids pressing those delicate buttons, because our reactions will not be the best, and they won't understand why. That reaction is the nature of the beast when you are tired and empty of good energy, so what we do is act from that place. How can that ever work out to be the best and loving in nature? Instead, we react with anger, we get emotional on the smallest thing, and we are tearful and shout out orders at them or become critical and blow things way out of proportion. And if you can't take it out on your kids, you will take it out on someone else—perhaps even yourself, going back to your self-deprecating self.

When kids challenge us, let it be. We need to learn to celebrate it and encourage them to communicate clearly and consistently. Both can learn to ask and respond with kindness and curiosity. Try to not misinterpret them because you are too busy and attached solely on your agenda with yourself or them. Take note, everyone here who are parents or teachers, as this can lead to unnecessary miscommunication, which will not help the relationships grow. We have touched on the impact of difficult relationships on health, and the consequences of that.

It is so frustrating that the majority of health debates are on what we eat and how much we exercise or not. People who eat well and exercise are still ill, have chronic illnesses, and in some cases, are worse off than people who are fat and therefore judged to be unhealthy. Ill health can get a hold on you from any angle that is out of balance, and we need to always think of the bigger picture and the root cause, and then pave the way to return to health in a joined and wholesome way. Healthy eating, nutrition, and exercise will not be the only dimensions that give us optimal health. There are other dimensions, like environment; and the status of all your relationships is another dimension; how fulfilled we live each day and so on. Like everything in our world, and now even more than ever—through the influence of social media and the access to all things shiny and bright, the wave of nutritionists and veganism, like flared jeans, once was a craze—so much attention has been on lifestyle and that healthcare professionals do not have nutritional knowledge, which is true, but it's not that. I am personally shaking my head at this fashionista approach because it misses something fundamental again. Your nutritionist may advise you to eat more vegetables or a certain type of fruit because it is shown to help with aspects of your health and recovery, so you go to the shops to get yourself everything on the list. The problem is, these days, in terms of their nutritional value, fruit or vegetables grown and eaten at source are very different from their equivalent that have been sitting on a refrigerated shelf in a supermarket. Teach them health in a new way, in a fully integrated way. Teach them what food is, and why eating more greens, fruit, legumes, grains, and meats are good for them. Explain and take the time to do that, invest in educating them about their bodies and what is important, and tell them how they can look after it simply. That is what is missing in health care education today. We don't get that information from outside, and we don't get it in our homes. Mothers are too busy to love themselves, let alone teach their daughters and sons how to do it. Some simply don't know and are just passing the racket around that was passed around to them, without re-evaluation or interruption. People try and push certain ways of eating, but people like to eat according to their culture, so it is about finding and nurturing a happy, refined balance, and opening people's minds and hearts to a different approach, if their approach is in fact making them ill. Learn from best practice, but again, it is not about one rule fitting all. As convenient as that may be, and many health practitioners try and sell you that convenience and illusion, it is just not true. Only you can individualise your health. It has to start with you and stay with you. It has always been simple, so why have we complicated it for ourselves? Because we are brainwashed and conditioned into submission and falseness.

Like I said, educate them on healthy eating, but go up a level and educate them on where their food comes from, what foods there are in world, what they look like, and what all the different herbs and spices are that add interest to food. Teach them about nutritional value in food, not just to count calories; in fact, there needs to be limited talk on counting calories in foods, but definitely knowledge on processed and packaged foods. Take them shopping and ask them to choose ingredients to make a meal from scratch. Teach them your specialties early on. If we all do our bit and stop buying the quantity of processed food, or meat from factory farms—cheap meat, sugar-laden products, and fizzy pop—each of us, little by little, will collectively make a difference to global health and our planet. I am due to revisit my country of birth, Tanzania, Africa, and I am nervous because I know how much infiltration will be evident from big food companies for processed junk. Even I know that places like that, and other countries with low and middle income that are developing fast, and rightly so, are being brainwashed by processed food manufacturers and suppliers. They are on the lookout for big profits because of its virgin territory through convenience and cost-effective living, thereby dangerously changing the health of those nations, just like in the West. My health, if I had lived there as a child growing up, would be better than the health of the children in the West, but not as good as it was back then, some 40 years ago. That makes me so sad and very angry.

Where nutrition is depleted, talk to them about proper supplementation. Let's face it; today, our food is not as good as before. The soil is over-farmed and depleted in nutrition, so if you can grow some vegetables in your garden, please teach them to do that.

Another classic dysfunctional mechanism for ill health is environment, which means our work, our homes, our towns and cities, and our schools. I have mentioned how these environments can go against our health and wellbeing, so be mindful of that as well. Make your home environment the best it can be in terms of health and wellness, especially when you have children around, because things can get quite cluttered, busy, and noisy, and you need to cultivate an environment where there are different zones in the home, where people can spend time being quiet and meditating. I think many people think that homes with these zones only belong to the rich; and yes, they may have big enough homes to be able to do this very distinctly, but even a small space can be converted. The important thing is to use those spaces, areas, or even structures within the home at appropriate times. You can create so much to have your home encourage wellbeing and wellness, and it does not need to follow any particular trend, like Zen living, or to make it into a sanctuary. The reason I want the home to be like this is because it is taking a lot longer to cultivate this in other environments not in your control, like the high street in your local town, which is packed with eating places and takeaway shops that are all just adding to ill health. Why would local council and public health support the rental of fish and chip shops, kebab shops, cake shops, burger joints, cigarette vape shops, or low-cost Poundlands selling mostly crap, all in the same line as each other? Surely, they have the capacity to balance what type of businesses go into the town centre's space, but they don't, as eating and food outlets make up a substantial local economy. So, with your home, think about and plan intuitively what the needs are of your busy family life. Return the dining table back to a centrepiece, where all eating can take place without any distractions apart from being together, and if you can extend this to an outside space into the garden or patio, even better.

I love alfresco dining, and I do it with my family as often as the British weather will allow me. Think about where you want your family to be together, to play, talk, and so on, and then where people can go for some solitude and restfulness.

Think about your work spaces and your work environment, which people are near you, and who is in your team—who are they really, and what personality is dominant? Any company too heavy with managers is not going to be ideal health wise. Why? Because they are puppets, and if the leadership is tricky, so will they be. The best way to think about if you are happy there or not, is if your values align with the company, and theirs with yours. Think about how much food is brought in and what types. You know that the NHS is given so much food by happy patients; staff are always chomping on chocolate, biscuits, and foods that are high in sugar and heavily processed. With so many nurses and doctors that are overweight themselves, is this ideal, along with long stressful working hours? Any environment that cripples human wellness and growth needs to be evaluated. This is one of the greatest risks and can lead to our demise. Your home environment has to be a harmonious balance between rest, curiosity, learning, activity, and human growth, but homes today are not restful.

There are some unique schools in the world that put their children first—their holistic approach for development, innocence, and wisdom, the energy of serving others in their quest to be successful— why can't this be the norm? Those same children not only have drive and determination, but they are also academically very successful. Why is our corporate world not paying more attention to human development, their doors only opening to a contact in a cautious way? The doors should be flung open to coaches and heart-centred practitioners, people who can really teach and guide, and have knowledge that is so important. It's life changing, but in reality, only the top most people who have wealth behind them gain access to it. The world is used to hierarchy and control. This is what breeds layers of poverty. It is the poverty of ignorance and lack of awareness.

Why are organisations paying so little attention to the wellbeing of their people, and if they do, why is it inconsistent and piecemeal? Why is more not being done? Resources are shafted somewhere into a marketing budget and training mundane, repetitive rubbish into people for the sake of training and PR—the so-called corporate hard skills. Yet again, it is a tick-box exercise. There are many like me who are asking these same questions because we want improvements, and success for everyone, not just the elite; we are daring to challenge the status quo and will keep striving for vision and innovation, and we will say NO to any system that clips our wings. It feels tiresome, mundane, and dry, and we feel trapped and will find the quickest way out of that environment because we know the difference between our resonance and dissonance. We are our own leaders and are not afraid of becoming masters of our own destiny, and because of that, we also know who and what we want in our lives.

My way of thinking means that I take risks even as a mother. I know the impact on my family if things go wrong, but I still take risks because I am confident that the environment and the people I spend my time in and around, have similar if not the same strengths, and we can cope with anything. We correct the gaps because we have the most powerful asset: our health. Our minds are healthy, and we can make decisions confidently and clearly. Our bodies can cope with short-term stress because we have fed and watered it well, and we have kept our need for action in motion and exercised. We believe wholeheartedly in better things. We have belief in ourselves and tremendous faith in the Universe, and in like-minded individuals and groups around the world.

What short-term challenges do for other people is that it kicks them off their horse, and they lie on the ground, not knowing how or when to get up, and sometimes they stay there, beaten and in denial. You have to be healthy to be able to respond quickly to anything life throws at you, no matter what it is. You, and only you, are in charge of your world. Make it a healthy one.

Teach them the values of holistic health from the day they are born, by modeling it in yourself and your partner, being very clear with grandparents, aunties, and uncles too, in terms of this clear goal. Explain and discuss with any weak links in the chain, and lift them up to better ways and health at the same time. Many people do what they do with food offerings because it makes them feel good about themselves. They don't think about the person being offered it. Interrupt that chain of thought and actions by opening their eyes in a kind, loving way.

It is the best thing you will ever do, next to having them in the first place. When they are old enough, then start discussions about a lifestyle that is about balance of health in spirit, body, and mind. Teach them to be positive, happy, and aware, and to manage their mind. Show them the difference between being lost and found, between dark and light, and the difference between finding their own answers and asking in the first place as they search. Teach them to be at one with themselves, not broken into pieces and glued on superficially just to show the world they have it together, when they really don't! We owe all this to the future generations, and in order to do this, we need to work on ourselves and start again if we have to. It is never too late to start, but what a start it is. There is time and hope for a better and more unified, happy world. It is time. Talk about health and wellness, and discuss all things that happen to us that contradicts that. Warn the little children on what to watch out for and what can be rewarded. Let's stop talking about illness and sickness. Let's change the focus, and work in harmonious partnership with each other rather than working only with people who position you well, or you them. There is huge value in sharing.

Question for you:
"What are you going to do about your health
from this day onwards?"

Guiding principle:
"Believe, think, and act on your health,
as it is the ultimate force for good."

Family Roles and Dynamics

Let me further share my upbringing to illustrate the points made here.

Firstly, what you need to understand is that families are fluid systems, and many things get passed back and forth through this structure. Any system offers duplicity and a copying process, and if something works well, it makes sense to pass it on. Sometimes outdated stuff also gets passed around. It is true that some do not steer away from this structure that essentially holds the family in place, but others in the family also use the flexibility to try out their own things, and this is particularly true if someone from a different culture or upbringing is included in the family structure. The mix and injection of something new is always welcome as long as the system can be flexible enough. There are some family systems where this is not the case, essentially locking youth in a very old way of being; and doing that can be crippling to them, and the fear of speaking out can be distressing. However, it is always good to welcome a mix in personalities, and not all need to be loud and outspoken. You will know that there are certain things you do or say that remind you of your parents' sayings and doings. We have taken those things on, and when it is time for that to come out, we get surprised and almost shocked that we did that or said this, perhaps to our children. In any case, it usually comes out when you least expect it, and if and when it does, that says that you took those kinds of thinking patterns, emotions, and behaviours on, perhaps subconsciously. It is natural and normal to take things on; after all, most of us spend a substantial time with our parents before we leave the roost, and even then the influence can still continue.

I have lived in two worlds my entire life: in the Indian world and in the modern Western world. It has its own unique experiences, and although challenging at times, it has been a rich and colourful tapestry of experiences.

What happens for some is that these beliefs become indoctrinated, and then they can't think for themselves, basically living a copy of their parents' lives. This can be okay in some cases but not in others. It becomes a wall they can't get past.

One of the biggest challenges for our elderly is that they can't let go of the past, and so they stay stuck there. Experiences of their NOW are therefore disappointing and hard. They feel like they don't belong in this world anymore, and this withdrawal and loneliness makes them ill, or they certainly see a decline in their health quite quickly, first through low mood, and finally through a physical manifestation of some disease that brings them nearer to death. It is true that even if they have a physical illness, if their mind and social interaction is kept strong and inclusive (i.e. they still have meaning, and they are not giving up), they will live longer and sometimes actually reverse illness despite their age. For our elderly, and also everyone else for that matter, interaction is critical to longevity and healthy living. It is our duty to keep our elders involved in the most meaningful ways in our lives, and also to encourage them to keep living according to their likes and desires.

Families also have a direct impact on what roles are given to individuals, and what conditional attributes they take on. Some examples here are labels and beliefs given, like "breadwinner," "boys don't cry," "girls are weaker than boys," and "your mother is the strong one in the family."

My experience with family roles was positive overall. What we allow and teach within the family setting is instrumental to how we learn to navigate life. My own parents were very different from many other folk in our family, and crafted a life that they loved; yet through my own reflections and clarifications, some of their inner beliefs, traditions, and customs were actually still quite limiting. The one that used to get me was the belief that "rich people are rogues," or "we can't be rich; it's not in our destiny," or "we are too nice, and people take advantage." So, I know that I am a nice girl and a proven businesswoman, but I always had that voice that kept saying that I was not anything special, and that I could not be rich or generate income in my business because I was not rogue enough, and being nice was an attribute that would not help me make a sharp businesswoman or money for that matter. How bizarre is that belief? The evidence was to the contrary: I was able to make money, generate income, and nurture my business to success, and all through being nice. I never stepped over anyone or positioned myself ahead of anyone by using people. I had the humbleness to help people by going the extra mile, and I was fully aware of all the sharks that wanted to take advantage, and today still do. I had my health though, but despite all this, I never really believed that I would make it in business or that it was meant to be. It could have been a self-fulfilling prophecy, but I changed the narrative in time. Today, I believe that people who are nice and put their heart into running a business are the ones that succeed, and there are plenty of very successful businessmen and women who are genuinely nice, because that does not mean not being sharp or being a good leader, or even having an eye for entrepreneurship and business. The point is that sometimes individuals in the family can pass on their struggles and their beliefs.

This belief was passed down from generations of the same thinking and is simply not true. You are what you believe, but without the knowledge of how they influence you, they can limit you your whole life, and new generations are being born into this kind of thinking. They find examples and experiences in life that match these beliefs and make them true, and then there is no way out unless they shift that thinking in a deep way, and dispute it by finding all the evidence against it that you also have experienced. Perhaps in history, many,

many generations ago, this belief may have been true, and the evidence they got was also true; but today, and in my generation, this is untrue. Looking back at the kinds of positions and jobs my family had—surprise, surprise—they were not in business but instead were very well recognised academics, medics, scientists, and teachers. Early on in my career, I also started out in academic science. My father was in business, and yet he came from an academic family background. He was a superb businessman, and he had the biggest heart. I learned from him in so many ways. He broke the mold and made his life his, and he wanted the same for my sister and me, and my mum too. Other family members were also very important to him, and that included all his brothers and sisters, his parents, and extended family, and his huge friendship circle that spanned all over the world. What he created was real wealth, not just in monetary form.

I have seen firsthand that many people with lots of money, rightly or wrongly made, are not blessed fully—they are ill, have broken marriages, suffer tragedy and controversy, and can be emotionally deficient, lacking love at some level and to a degree. That is not wealth. So perhaps having the belief that nice people can be anything they want and are helped by bigger things, is a good one to hold.

I have known and worked with many, where their experience of parents was very negative, to the point that many of them had fallouts and no longer spoke to them in a way that was healthy and genuine, and as much as they convinced themselves that they didn't care anymore about what happened to their parents, they did find that there was a gap in their life. They had sadness, regret, and disappointment, and had no way to put it right; and someone, despite their sadness, still felt it was not what they wanted. Some would interact with their parents in the most minimal way by carrying out duties, but in a resentful way and talking behind their backs on how inconvenient that was. I found this so sad that they could not let go, and I am a firm believer that any relationship, no matter how bad, can be repaired to the point of giving peace to all concerned, even if it does mean parting with dignity. The disharmony they carried around with them was affecting their physical health, their emotions, and minds, and there was no sense of peace or pride.

The interesting commonality, when they were asked what had caused the demise of the relationships with a parent or parents, was the response that they had overly critical parents who never listened and loved in a way that felt authentic.

For example, many feared their father for being very stern and critical, so they learned to only fit in a way that pleased their fathers or with men that had that trait, and not what they really wanted to do or say, and they never took risks or lied, because they would only be found out and get punished. Many mentioned how fear led their lives, and how clever and creative they had to become in order to not be found out when they did anything that would be considered bad or controversial. Taking risks is something we all have to do; otherwise, we live out our lives being sheltered, only controlling what we know, and never quite experiencing anything new, and never really developing faith and trust in our own potential.

We know that it is good for children to take risks so that they learn skills. Many felt that it was only after they left home that they could really start living, but during those break-free years, the damage had already been done, and the safety and familiarity of that way of an upbringing meant that they would get hooked up with similar types of role models in managers, colleagues, and even marital partners, who also were overly critical, and they would become trapped again, living their lives fearfully rather than courageously.

The more we come away from roles, and act instead in union with each other, helping and encouraging the best versions of each other, no matter what our circumstances are, we will be stronger, happier, and more united. Children do that, so why can't we maintain that?

So I invite you to think of all the things that work like this, and also the things that don't work for you in your family, and come to grips with the mess, even if it feels like you want to ignore it. Start with an open discussion and a good intention for a stronger bond with each other; forgive yourself and everyone for all the mistakes they made, and start to be guided by the best version of yourself. You know what feels healing and fabulous, so speak the truth and be authentic.

I absolutely love my culture. I am an open-minded and Hindu. There are so many good things about being both. We have so much that goes into relationships that encourage peace and harmony with each other. I am finding that Indians now living under other influences are the ones going astray, and I feel real gratitude that I had and have the wisdom to integrate good practices from my culture, but also to open my heart to other cultures without any detriment to me and my family, even if others cannot do the same to me.

Question for you:
"What are the conflicts that exist in your life, if any,
where on reflection, it is time to move on from?"

Guiding principle:
"We are all meant to be part of something bigger than we are; the
Universe moves us around so that we can experience it."

Learn from Each Other, Collectively and Globally

Think about what you have been taught that has had a profound effect on your life, and how important that teaching was. What if you were never taught it, ever? Have you shared that teaching with anyone else?

How much was related to health in you? My vision is for everyone to teach health in the same capacity: an overarching subject matter that is taken seriously rather than being stumbled across because you need to see a health practitioner, or because you have settled all the kids and now you can finally look after yourself. How many people think this way and say it? What if the lack of health was the key to all our problems of the world? It is when it's out of balance. For example, extremism in any form is a lack of balanced thinking; it is crooked and all or nothing, severely aligning the thinking path with extreme resentment and anger.

If balance was that easy to ascertain, do you think we would be where we are? Look at our planet, our countries, poverty and our economy, governments, the rate at which disease is increasing globally, and the unjust distribution of wealth. Something needs to change, don't you think? The problems we have in the world are co-created, but let's become better people. Let's stop blaming others, and instead take action and step up for the causes that are our passions, and which are for the greater good. We are, after all, the cause and effect.

We know how inadequate health provision is in some countries; however, there are healthier people in poorer and simpler lands than in the Western and richer countries. Sure, many people die of snake bites, accidents, and lack of good food and clean water, but they are still so humble and don't moan; they fully accept their way of life whilst hoping for a better way for their children and future families. When someone comes along and gives them an opportunity for education or hope, they grab it, and the light in their eyes is sheer beauty. They value life. Compare that to someone who has everything and yet values nothing. Look at our young nowadays, lighting fires to trees in public places, or plotting to kill people at the age of ten, and yet they have food, a home, and the opportunity of free education. They just lack meaning and positive fulfillment, and faith of any sort. Their spirit is stuck in a box, yearning to be let out and be free. It's trapped in the closed mindset. They must be helped.

We are lucky that we have the NHS in the UK, yet so many abuse it. I am motivated to have my health and be free of any medical intervention in the way of pharmaceutical drugs or treatments for preventable chronic illnesses. I value the NHS and all the staff that work in it. I am so lucky to have a healthcare system designed to help me when I do get sick or have an accident, and I feel safe if I do have to go. I have the confidence that the doctors and nurses that could potentially look after me are good people and want to provide an exemplary level of care. But just because I live in the UK, it is not my right to use the doctors' time for unnecessary illnesses caused by smoking, or drinking so much that I can't stand up on a Saturday night. What if the NHS stopped treating people who are so hell bent on mistreating themselves that they waste valuable resources and put pressure on the system that should be valuing the people that look after themselves? It will not be easy to turn a blind eye, but if we do, perhaps health will become even more valuable, and people will make the effort to look after themselves better and make better choices. When something is given freely, its potential to be abused rises, and that opportunity, for some, is greater than in others.

We live under an illusion, a fantasy that the NHS is free and that our health is their problem, but we pay over the odds in taxes for it; so no, it is not free. Meanwhile, a healthy family struggles to eat properly because their tax bill keeps increasing every year to essentially pay for the lack of responsibility of someone else. How is that fair and just? It's not nice to hear the truth, but the people who deny the truth really know their truth. If we don't take responsibility for ourselves, how can we change the distribution of wealth and other natural resources, and make it pleasant for every living person and creature?

It is pointless to sit on the sidelines and wait for some magic pill that will make everything right for you in an effortless way.

We need to prioritise health amongst other things that we also want—it's linked. It does not have to be yes- but, that rolls off the tongues of many. It cannot be traded for anything else; but in reality, it is traded all the time for chasing more money, wealth, and someone else's ideals.

I am not in favour of paying high taxes to support a broken and less than empowering healthcare system, or any other broken public service that does not service people. I would prefer to be giving that money to charitable causes, diminishing poverty, helping homeless people, getting children revised and updated education that they deserve, and putting money into genuine research and innovation. That is a way in which I decide where and what I earn, and what it goes toward.

With consistent health behaviours, thoughts, and actions, we can teach and guide people to be just as effective as we are, with some wiggle room to make it their own. If we all did it, even in a small way, and be consistent with it, imagine how different your world could be. I always remember, when traveling to poorer countries, what they would say to me when I told them where I was from. Once they knew it was the UK, their response was: "Oh yes, people who are rich, fat, and sick!" I did not take offense, probably because I was not any of those things at that time, but I got it, and sad to say, I agree. Let's all change this narrative and the perception of us, not because they could then approve of us, but because it gives us a good reality check.

So let's get clear on how we can include health in our daily lives, what we can think and say, and how we can make sure that we action what is necessary for us to stay in good health. My motivation is to never be reliant on drugs, and to keep all my organs in optimal working order. Once you know what you are motivated to do, you can plan what needs to be put into place to serve this aspect of your life.

When I meet people, sometimes for the first time, it is easy to discuss some other aspect of their life, but when we come to discussing health, they suddenly have to leave; or if people get to know what I do, they are too afraid to have any conversation on health, just in case they get found out—so many live a lie when it comes to their health. I want a world where people can openly discuss how well they are or how ill they are, without sounding like a broken record. If you had health in the way I want for you, you could not keep it from anyone; it would be oozing out of you, and the energy you would bring to the world, and your own world, would be miraculous. But alas, people are weary of an open heart. In today's world, people that are genuine and goodhearted are not recognised, and people can be weary of them, labelling them as not to be trusted. Our world is so disconnected that shallow people and narcissistic people are celebrated and popularised. We don't really know goodness when it presents itself; it is not always a trusted attribute. We still have so much racism, prejudice, elitist attitudes, and discrimination and judgement, when actually we are all connected just by being part of the most unique of species—our human race.

Humans copy each other, so if your habits and sources of thoughts and behaviours toward health are no good, then it will be passed on and copied in more ways than you think are possible. We are really a giant photocopying race, so surely we have a responsibility to each other that only good things get copied, and that we strive to easily correct the "not serving us" traits, without fear of rejection or unfriendliness. Health is a duplicable system in its basic rights, but people don't even embrace the basics, and that's the problem. It has to start from the beginning AGAIN.

We can give permission to ourselves and others at this time to become more confident in our health, and as long as it is from an informed place, the debate that takes place on health and other important progressive topics is so much fun and is actually enlightening. We all know someone in our lives that needs help, and we can open up conversation easily and openly, and not wait for the right time, place, or environment. Just dive in—name the truth!

We all know how we tread on eggshells around a family member when there is an illness we feel sorry for! You know, it may seem the right thing to do, to avoid hurting them, or to promote controversy or conflict, but being brave and courageous is the way you open their eyes by talking about it, or they will sink into a deeper hole with their illness and would not be able to see or feel their own strength inherent in them to get themselves out of it. When someone talks of illness, listen to them up to a point, and when you know they are sinking past that initial level, talk instead on what they want, and how healthy they can be and once were. Keep mindful of their best life and what they can still be. That's what will get them recovering and resolute to heal. Don't add fuel to their downhill spiralling. The trick is to know the balance and timing between empathetic listening and empowerment.

Most people also may know that in such circumstances as cancer, diabetes, bereavement, or mental illness in a family, it is a challenge to know what to say and how to behave, and any guarded approach to skirt round issues of their failing health are intuitively felt by the person suffering the illness, so you may as well just name what is going on for you to get them engaged in your discussions. They will open up. Tell them how you feel, that you are scared and worried for them, and ask them what they need or even want. You have to renegotiate the terms of your relationship during such bouts of illness that impact more than just them. Perhaps they want a visionary that injects hope into them to say that they can fight it and get better, even if initially they don't believe you. Eventually they know that they don't want to be a burden; they want hope and answers. Name and show concern from a sincere place, and discuss solutions; think of their motivation. There is nothing worse than someone who is ill and wants to get better, who has the strength not to be defeated by their illness, and you come along and tell them not to have false hope! You just pulled the wire from the life support machine, and it flat lined.

You don't have to be a doctor to save lives.

So, instead, offer your full attention. I am not asking you to be god; just be sensible and informed, and hold the torch of hope, health, and wellness for you and them. We get what we focus on. That's the universal law!

If we focus on sickness, we get sicker. Let's focus on wellness in every human around the world. We have work to do because we have focused on sickness far too long for the gain of those elitist— remember them, that small but very controlling number of people who have been playing with our health as though we were puppets on a string. That system has focused on sickness, lack, and depravity, and uses control.

It is wrong, and we are heading in the wrong direction with our health, but there is hope, and there is a small and sincere army around the world: doctors who uncover the truth, holistic practitioners, spiritual healers, life coaches, children with their innocence and wisdom, and the closest form of God, and YOU. We are gathering pace to correct this abuse, and together we will correct things.

For me, I am here to make you turn around, and together we can create a collective momentum in all of our wellbeing.

Question for you:
"We are nearing the end of this book,
so what have you learned? Make a list at this point,
and you can read it over and then elaborate on it later."

Guiding principle:
"Our main purpose is one of self-discovery,
and mastery of mind, body, and heart; then to teach it to everyone
we come across, to the best of our ability."

Chapter principle:
"Communication about your desire for health and the health of others, has to be from day one. It has to be integrated with life every single moment. Be your own leader, take full ownership, and make it an essential part of your daily living."

Chapter 10
The Future Vision

Just Imagine

I would like you to go somewhere quiet and peaceful, with no interruptions for at least 10–15 minutes. Please read these instructions so that you know what you are going to do. Please set a timer if you need to; that will help you relax and not keep watching the time, especially if you are new to quietening your mind and visualising. Please ask others not to disturb you. You can pass it on to others in your household after you experience the peace and calming energy that comes over you.

Once there, set your alarm if you wish, and then put your phone down and away from you. If you are looking at the sea, at flowers or trees, or at a beautiful picture or family portrait, from wherever you have gone to, look at it in front of you in a relaxed, appreciative manner for a few minutes whilst taking deep breaths in and out. Now close your eyes and continue taking deep breaths slowly in and out. After 7 breaths, with your eyes still shut, say this affirmation, and only this one: "I am my best self, my higher self, and my health is divine." Repeat this affirmation each time, saying it more and more with your whole heart, and feeling its effect more and more each time you say it. About 7 times is good, if you can get there, and if you have gone past that, then that's fine.

You should have a few minutes left for this as well that way. Now stay there in this space, literally, and if any other thoughts come in contrary to the above affirmation, just try and ignore them, but don't fight them. Just be passively aware of them but don't focus on them. Just focus on the quiet, peaceful silence. Do this until the timer rings, and then slowly open your eyes, get your balance, and then read this final chapter.

Optimal health in all of us is the way forward for greater and best balance in the whole world. We will think better, do better, and feel better, and we will be more united. Health will be equal and will not depend on how wealthy you are. We are all the same in terms of the basic and inherent workings of our minds and bodies. It is only our learning and conditioning that separates us in groups according to our ability, potential, and wealth. Without health, we will be torn in ourselves, and therefore collectively torn, leaving gaps to fuel extremism, pessimism, and a divided world, where very few have the best. It is only the commitment we make to ourselves in restoring and protecting a healthy mind, body, and spirit that will give us all the tools and pure desire to do good for each other and truly come up with creative solutions for advancement in our world. If we don't value our own bodies and minds, how can we value it in others?

Why should we strive for innovation? How can we pray for health and wealth when we don't actually live it ourselves? For those who have it and know they have it, don't get all proud about it and judge others that you think are beneath you. Help raise them up to your level or greater. When you have a healthy mind, body, and spirit, you just could not put yourself above any other human, no matter what and who they are. So you still may have work to do. I am further along, and I still have work to do.

We are not born with discipline, only survival instincts. We have to create our own discipline by learning of its benefits, and in health, as you now know, it is vital. Be under no illusion that your health belongs in someone else's hands; it's yours at the start, in the middle, and at the end. It does not matter what your experience of life is; acknowledge it fully, make peace with it, and move on. Some of the strongest and healthiest people in the world have limbs missing or have only one kidney. They did not give up or give in. They learned how to accept whatever life had thrown at them. They will never understand the reasons for their pain, and should not try to, but they did keep strong in their mind and heart by appreciating, accepting, surrendering, and taking risks to keep moving up higher, and to be happy and grateful that they are alive and that this was meant to be. If you are someone who thinks that every bad situation you face is someone else's fault, wondering why you are victim of what life has thrown at you and how unfair it is, you will get stuck there; but if you are here, ready to accept it, that's brilliant, and you may need a little help to get you going. It's your choice—make it better and make it differently, but always with sincere love for yourself.

By challenging the best in others, whether they want it or not, is not being interfering. If meant and felt with complete purity and sincerity, it is a gift to transform life and to enhance it upwards toward the greater good. Do that for yourself and others.

We will again become united as a human race. Without it, we will feel resentful, envious, and unbalanced, and we will have too many victims of life. Imagine our planet then. Can these people ever have a vision for a better planet, people, and prosperity?

We have come a long way, and there is better in the world than the means with which bad stuff gets all the exposure. Let's change that. We have been brainwashed enough by the media on how they want us to see the world whilst goodness is truly lost. Let's report that instead.

I want our world to be fairer, more equal, and diverse, where people understand and accept our cultural inheritance and differences in the way we choose to live, but ultimately, and what transcends way higher, is that we are all the same in spirit, and those who are lost can find their way back the minute they choose to. They have to desire it, and until they are ready, we cannot impose, but we continue to talk to them in a good way. I want a disease-free world as much as is possible. I want normal people—the underdogs—to shine out and be given a voice of change. I want complete change in our working lives and education systems. I need your help, and to start now for the sake of humanity, our young, our unborn, and Mother Earth. There is no superior person in the human race, but we can all be a superior human being with our health intact.

Perhaps that may be what unlocks the part of the brain that is still asleep and is not used; maybe that's our next evolutionary ascent, but the passport to that are good people, and more importantly, awakened and self-realised people. There are many already, but the collective voice is not together, so it gets lost with the noise of wars, abuse, and ill health. Whilst that process gets the attention, we are not seen or heard enough or taken seriously enough, and more importantly, valued enough. Many more, I know, seek it, and it is just a matter of time before we gather to create a positive and uplifting force to be reckoned with.

Why develop robots to do our work; that's a sure straight line to our extinction. We need each other, to connect with each other, no matter how small and insignificant the task is. Robots are being created to replace human jobs because of money, efficiency, and sometimes greed. Yes, it's wonderful to see human intelligence taking things to the next level, but too much intelligence, and lack of wisdom and heart, can destroy.

In order for us to be truly united, we have to unite ourselves first. We have to become one with ourselves, seek our higher purpose, and do better for mankind everywhere. Start at home, increase your range to your friends and family, and to your local community and social groups. You are your job!

So close your eyes and imagine that you and all your loved ones are healthy, happy, free, and peaceful, and yet energetic and in harmony, enjoying and protecting our world together, doing what you love and being a testament to your inner values. It's beautiful, isn't it?

Question for you:
"How was that space and time for you,
when saying that affirmation?"

Guiding principle:
"We are better than any force that tries to darken us.
Our eyes see light."

Conditioning for a Brilliant World and Future

Our primitive brains are what they are, and there is a part of the brain that likes familiar conditioning systems. We do have our higher brain, and in order for us to learn a wholly new way of life, where health is fully integrated in a way that you and your family are not familiar with, you will need to bypass those areas of your brain that keep you small and comfortable. You are not in danger, so it does not need to dictate survival patterns. Work with creativity and vision, and where your true potential is.

We have an even more powerful subconscious mind, which is where most of what we do and experience drives us, without us knowing what's in charge there. It's a silent and most powerful part of our minds, and is still not fully understood properly. This is where our unconscious drivers to our thoughts, emotions, and behaviours are functioning, and our human challenge is to understand ourselves properly and deeply, to become self-aware. Our job is to master our minds, where we notice how we think, and to stop that thought in its track and change it to a better thought, even when our buttons are being pressed and life can feel drab.

It is a process that many people shy away from through fear of not liking what they may find. I say that if you fear it, you know that about yourself, so why protect the bits you don't like—let them go and seek a better way. To change this, make it a habit, and do it consistently and make an imprint in your subconscious mind by adding in affirmations.

Therefore, you need to reframe today for your tomorrow, and whoever you work with or come across, or if you are about to have children, reframe health in a way that will serve you all your life as a way forward. Convince yourself that you have the best health today (even though you may not), and work on your health as if it was optimal today. If that was the case, would you eat that second packet of crisps? Would you say no to a buddy who wants you to run with him? Would you say no to your body's signs of needing sleep? Would you override any of your body's signs and symptoms, and the intelligent feedback it gives you?

That is how you start making the change. Too many people make excuses. I get it; I used to be that person, and I am far from perfect, but my imperfections and ever-evolving self is the founder of this book, my health vision, and intention for you. I am able to get a grip and act with courage during difficult times. Imagine being in the company of awakened, enlightened, and optimally healthy people. It is so energising and motivating, and the feeling of wellness is first class. Communication is so easy and transparent, and people are genuinely sincere and kind here.

For too long, we have sold our own health to unethical people who seek to cut corners, misinform us, and control us. Why would I, or you for that matter, give your health away to people like that, whose policies benefit them directly, and their small but close circle of colleagues.

Why? There is no logical answer, and if you asked them personally, they would not know either, because they are part of a system in part corrupt and tailored to profit only by ill health, and they remain the ignorant party, quite oblivious to any wrong doing or even actually looking for the truth. We, on the other hand, can wake up to it, make a stand, help those who know it but have no wings to fly out of the hole they are trapped in, or we simply can ignore it for an unhealthy life, and trust the perpetrators who are invisible from our view. So instead, we trust accessible people on the ground and front-facing— our health care providers and grocery brands. They may be perceived as intelligent and members of society that are important, vital even, but that does not make them want the best for you or me either. So take a reality check here, and listen to your own intelligence, using your mind, body, emotions, and spirit—your whole self!

Say NO to these that keep company and collude to ill health, in this closed circuit of agriculture, food, and unethical healthcare and government, and take charge of your own way. Research, find out the real deal, and evaluate what's right for you. Look, if you need a diagnosis, go see a medical practitioner, but don't then just take a prescription and their advice, and run to the drug store and get your drugs and start on them. Has the full story for your ailments, aches, and pains been evaluated, or are you just a textbook case and are labelled because your collective signs and symptoms seem to point to this or that? Remember, all human brains look for and like familiarity and rationality with what fits in nice neat boxes, and doctors' brains are not wired any differently. Many in our public services are used to running with one-way directives. Challenge your GP in a way that drives their intelligence to do better and to be better, and to offer healthcare in the way it was meant to be offered, human to human, which allows for a two-way discussion on all choices. I would like to see the medical profession less prescriptive and more exploratory. I would like to see science become more creative. This in itself will revive the tired doctors, because it will connect them back to the desire to actually heal and help their patients in more ways than they do now. Our brains are designed to be stimulated for life; let's give them the right challenges, and the correct measures of stress and new learning to do this. We like problem-solving tasks. We can think higher. And we are capable of making things that are complex, simple again.

If we are to encourage a whole future generation into valuing life and therefore health, then we need to take charge for what we give out and take in, and continuously work on self-development and learning to evolve more and more powerfully to pass on to the next generations. We spend so much time passing on our wealth, homes, cars, material possessions, and stocks and shares, and yet we ask ourselves if there is something more lasting and more powerful that we can pass on—the legacy of a healthy mind, body, and spirit. To pass that on, confidently, we need to ensure that we have what is right to pass on. I have worked with so many young people who have thankfully sought help because they did not want to be like mum and dad or any authority figures. They understood how much impact those ways and voices were having, and they did not want that. They mentioned examples of a no-risk taker type mum and dad, always being too careful on spending or taking risks in their lives while truly being embedded in their comfort zone, and then having a child who grew up and decided to go traveling to remote parts of the world, or to go into business and apply for a £20,000 loan from the bank.

The experience of these young people was the careful articulation of fear-based support. They lost clarity, vision, purpose, and eventually any fulfillment and aliveness in their lives. That's the impact on some people who are fighting for their cause and can't get the people to believe in them because of fear—it's crippling. This goes on for generations until someone breaks the status quo and interrupts the process. It is literally like pulling the cord when a train is in full speed.

Do you hear the shock, the shaking, the alarm, the sound of braking at high-speed metal on metal—the unheard sounds of people fearing for their safety and identity, shaken to the core—the wake-up call in many ways! Be the person who pulls the cord!

Let's challenge the status quo with our standard health practice. If you are good at it, don't keep it a secret; share it, teach them, and guide them to be better in their wellbeing. Let's ramp it up together for us all to enjoy life fully. Let's move away from unnecessary suffering and lifestyle disease, and concentrate on wellbeing and wellness.

Question for you:
"What is your experience of healthcare?"

Guiding principle:
"Get off this train that takes you round and round with your health,
always delivering to the same place, where nothing changes and
all you do is lose precious time given to you."

A Long Healthy Life

It's great that we are living longer around the world. We are of course richer in resources and opportunities—for work, business, and career; technology; medicine; clean water and food—that contribute to this. It's great to see our elders on the web, with mobiles, texting their grandchildren and family members with uplifting quotes and messages. I know my mum does, and she is not from a generation that had any enhancements or knowledge with technology that we have today, in terms of connecting to people and getting things done in a way that allows us to do it all from the comfort of our homes. She, like I do, still prefers face-to-face interactions; that social aspect is so much richer in my view. As you know from earlier chapters, this social interaction is crucial for a prolonged life of quality health. So as much as we can embrace technology and the instant gratifying ways to get things done in less time, we need to hold out on the quality of our social interactions. All we need is regular and consistent ways of connecting with people, whether that is saying hello to a stranger collecting his morning paper, or having a conversation with your neighbours as you catch them doing a little bit of gardening. One thing I do is to qualify how many people I have spoken to on a daily basis, and if I made a difference to someone, including myself, in some small way—smiling and saying hello is all that is required. I try to smile at everyone I come across, and say hello, despite the majority never quite returning the gesture as they pass by. I know that's quite sad, but don't get disheartened by it; people are of course wrapped up in their lives so much more than they even know. The important thing is that you do it.

You will be surprised that you could have a house full of people, family, and kids, and still feel lonely, because you hardly speak to them in a way that is meaningful and set with the intention of sharing love. Loneliness can wear you down, and wear your health down. Please connect to people always, through your entire life. That does not mean keeping busy with social stuff all the time; solitude and time to recharge is crucial. A balance and a dance between the two go a long way to a prolonged way of life.

A cardiologist friend explained to me that he can save patients from dying these days, who would historically have not survived a heart attack. He treats people with chronic heart disease, where he is able to prolong their lives with medical treatment and interventions that did not exist or were not as sophisticated as they are today; but despite this, there is a worsening of his patients' quality of life. They live in fear that one day their hearts will give out, and that the intervention is just borrowed time. It is, and they live on egg shells. He says that many patients live in fear of that happening, so they cannot ever be free, not like before their heart health let them down.

They experienced something that could have been fatal, and that in itself keeps them locked into the experience again and again—there is no escape from it. For family who don't have to say goodbye and feel grief any sooner or any longer than necessary, they will of course encourage any intervention to keep their loved one alive for longer, even with a great deal of compromise. For the patient, it seems that slow and eventual death, and the feeling that they are in a strait jacket, sometimes can be worse than death itself. They carry the burden, the risk of another heart attack or progressively declining health, and their life has to be adapted to the point that it is not free. Many become depressed and lose hope, feeling that they are locked in with no escape—the only escape being death itself. Can you imagine living a life without the freedom that only exists when you have your whole health? Is it not better to stay well and use more preventative methods to uphold your ultimate freedom? When you are burdened with ill health, do you not pray for a miracle or even a day without any problems? Suddenly then, you understand the value of good health.

Waking up every day with renewed vigour and vitality, being excited and having the energy to make every day count, is what quality of life is about. From this place, how valuable are you in work, as a parent, within other life roles, and with yourself? Just like little children who wake up every day dancing in the moment of a new day, with curiosity as if it was a holiday every day, having the freedom with our thinking and our time and the people who we choose to be with, we can all have this, and we can co-create a better world from this place, and even if you are here already, then think of what else is also possible.

Think about your quality of life with the analogy of cooking a meal: When you are excited to do it, and do it with love, using the best, freshest ingredients, your creation is delicious, but when you cook this meal as if it's a chore, or like you don't want to or you are angry, it does not turn out to be the best, does it? Carefully understanding your motivation to aspects of your health is essential. Give your health all the love it deserves.

So start by firstly rating your quality of life today, your health from the inside, and your energy. How are you? How do you feel? Don't lie to yourself; really think of what is great about it, what's missing, and how you would want your life to be. What's stopping you from being your best self? What are your obstacles? Are they real or fictional? Imagine that you have dealt with your obstacles, or have just put them out of your way and ignored them, and you can see a clear path in front of you—where would that path be taking you in your life and true desire?

Write the emotions you are feeling, and the thought you are thinking whilst you walk down this path. Who will be with you, and what will you be sharing with them? Please reflect on this and give yourself enough uninterrupted time to do this exercise. I would love to know what your experience was like in this, so please get in touch, on any of my social media channels through www.SanjayaPandit.com and write a comment under the hashtag #mybestlife.

Question for you:
"Think of a time when you felt completely free
so that you could do anything, anywhere, anytime;
you were light and bouncy, energetic, and just awesome."

Guiding principle:
"You deserve a long, healthy life. This body of yours... that's it!"

A World Free from Dis-ease

Anything that gives life, protects it, and has the capacity of restoring it, has to be a good thing. I am sick of the world paying an unbalanced amount of attention and focus on ill health, disease, death, tragedy, and people hurting each other and abusing life on our planet, and keeping each other sick. Until we are made aware of what's really going on, we will not use our eyes and ears and action the much needed change with our voices, hands, and feet. Our world population is increasing, and we are living much longer, and although nature has its own way of increasing its resources to sustain us, sometimes it is forced to act in ways that are devastating to the lives of innocent people. We are destroying its intentions for us all. It therefore struggles to sustain balance for longer and replenish us. It is only when we stop interfering with it, and trust it by being mindful of all the resources given to us, that it will help overall, and our own health will be better for it. It troubles me that we still have a lack of water and food in some parts of our global world, and then we have so much food being mindlessly wasted by the overconsumption in other parts of the globe. If we all just bought less, just sufficient enough for our true needs, and not be greedy, I know we would be healthier in ourselves and in global natural resources, and then we could bring equality to parts of the world that so badly need it.

Our news reports are consistently back to back with reports on tragedy, and how our actions have destroyed so much of our natural resources through greed and selfish control. And through the addition of accessible social media, we are now under assault from overload, being exposed to it 24/7. Notice how people get jittery when they are simply just waiting for the bus or meeting a friend, and they face just a few moments of nothing, and they have to dig their phone out because staying in the moment is so difficult these days. Instead of using those few precious moments of just *being*, they start *doing* by checking messages and re-reading old messages, nipping onto Twitter or Facebook, and scrolling through their timeline. It's a beautiful chance given to them to connect and bring themselves in the moment—that place of conscious, thoughtless awareness. Think about it: that space where you are fully aware of everything around you but have no thought—it's utterly peaceful and beautiful—true yoga.

I take great pleasure in meeting friends, and of course I will check my phone to see if they are okay and on their way; but once I know that,

I put it away and bring myself into the moment. I take in my surroundings, watch and smile at other people, and sometimes meeting an old friend who is running late has allowed me to make a new friend, someone who was just there, like me, being in the moment. If I had my head in my phone, scrolling through information, I would have missed that. So put your devices down and connect with people around you, and with the environment—the shapes, colours, and smells around you. It's a time to connect with yourself and check in with yourself; it's a chance to shut your eyes and go inwards for a few minutes. I would love for young people to know the value of this instead of calling it old fashioned living. Little do they know, they are slaves to their devices; and sadly, so is anyone that has a smart phone. There is a time and place for everything, but information overload is not on my agenda for health. The innovation of convenience through some technology is harmful.

It is already showing impact on our mental health, and on the health of our young people's minds. I see more and more young people who cannot communicate to their friends and family members in a way that is open, honest, and expressive. Their language, spelling, and sentence building skills suffer, and so do their thinking skills and cognitive skills with predictive text, as well as interpersonal skills, because they text so much or email, rather than talk. They also have little attention skills and are terrible at listening. They are always in such a hurry, as if they can't stand speaking anymore—it's a foreign language to them. Our younger generation can't talk to each other; they don't have the thought process or patience. The concern is that some of these will become important influential people, or maybe their potential may just decrease as they get wrapped up in this way of life!

I love gadgets and technological innovations, and that in itself is not the problem, but it's the way we are managing our time with it and without it. The advances we have made have transformed so many industries, and the concept of businesses being without technology would be crippling in their growth. This phase is growing very fast, so keeping up with it can be tiring and confusing. There is a flip side to anything, and we have to be able to use our intelligence to understand when we take technology too far, when we can embrace it, and when it is valuable to us.

Parents and teachers have to work harder in getting kids to engage face to face, have a discussion, solve problems, feel better about themselves, and action a balance between rest and a working practice. In fact, parents struggle with this, so how can they teach their children?

This unruly impact will be worse if something is not done about it now. It has to be now! I want to see a world and all its human inhabitants restore balance for themselves, and then share that impact with other living co-inhabitants. It is only when you feel well, really well, that you automatically seek to do better for yourself and others, to have a better state of being, be in harmony with yourself and nature, in a selfless way and one with complete awareness and mindfulness to go on to live a meaningful, fulfilling, and purposeful life. It is here that your productivity and creative skills are best and can take you to a whole new level in your life.

Nature knows how to balance. We do too, as we are part of nature if we let ourselves be that, but we don't. Our ego, pride, and mind state get in the way of that, whereas trees, for example, don't have an ego, or a watch for that matter, and as part of nature, they know how and when to shed their leaves and when to regrow and flower. It is in their blueprint, and anything that interferes with their blueprint will not allow this natural process. As humans and natural beings, we also have these inbuilt skills. As you know, we are always in our own way, and then that impacts us so that we are also in other people's ways. Would it be so bad if humans did what they did many years ago: listen to the cues from the environment; for example, when to rise early and when to sleep, and what to do with our time in between? We still had families, taught our kids things, and worked, so why is it so difficult to fit it all in today? What happens in tribal lands? When it gets dark, we tend to quieten down and go to sleep, not open a bottle of wine, give yourself acidity issues, and then try and get a good night's sleep. It won't happen! Is that intelligence or sheer stupidity? And by the way, I am not judging people who do that; but if you do, don't expect your health to be at its best. It is a choice again, like everything.

We are just about as far as we can be from our natural states as human beings.

It is time for resurrection and rebirth without physical death.

We have to manage our minds to keep focused on the good, the good in everything, including in us; and we can't see good in anything else until we see it in ourselves. It has to be true, genuine, and meant sincerely. I don't mean those happy-clappy events that superficially make you feel happy, and then, 24 hours later, it fizzles out and you are back to reality. Instead, how about knowing who you are, inside and out, and what's authentic and robust about you, your true desires and passion for living a life being optimised, changing your beliefs and paradigms from a place of awareness and knowledge, and looking and experiencing everything with renewed energy and vigour?

Or are you someone who is working only to retire, and in the meantime, get really old in your attitude to life?

I keep the company of people who don't want to ever retire; they love what they do, and each day they experience things with renewed vigour. The people and company they keep are with people like that, and they feed and nurture off each other energetically. Here, there is no harm in enjoying some good food and wine.

Are you around people like that, or around ones that keep watching the time—"When does the weekend start?" "How long till I retire?"—

saying no to everything that challenges them, because they are not paid enough to do that job, or are you around people who love what they do, what they are born to do, and are fulfilled and passionate life-giving people. Wherever you are, you have a choice to jump and step up, or continue on a flat line that feels like forever in time. Get yourself into a position to truly be alive, to be happy and joyous, and to live "dis-ease free."

Question for you:
"How can you make a contribution to a dis-ease-free world?"

Guiding principle:
"Life is so precious; breathe it in with your eyes wide open,
your ears fully listening, and your heart fully responsive."

Legacy for Health

By definition, legacy means "an amount of money or property left to someone in a will, or something left or handed down by the predecessor." The problem here is that you either have to die or you give it away, so it is no longer yours. My vision for a legacy for health is not a hand-me-down but an experience that is lived every day. It is that living and interconnectedness that gives a whole new meaning to legacy—your guidance, teaching, effectiveness, and proactive daily ways that are so beautiful, clear, and joyous that you impact not just one or a few but a mass, and in time, generations to come. It is so huge and so simple, and yet we are still to get started. We are stuck and going backwards into the darkness with our health. I have been a witness to discussions with people who don't understand why we are so unhappy, sick, fat, and pale in the West. They can't understand why we are like this, despite being wealthy and rich and having it all—in their eyes anyway! It's a great point they make, don't you think? The tide for wanting to live in the West is diminishing, certainly for people who truly understand about what quality of life means without the material handcuffs that we can be tied into. There is a real need to free our spirits and souls, and the liberty and happiness that comes with it. The East is very attractive to many, and even if they can't live there, many want to have the wisdom and knowledge on how to live that way of life, at least to some degree.

This legacy of health is the absolute reason to change our present health, our learnings, and gifts from the past; and it's the integration into the start of our present and future health, so that every single one of us can empower each other for best and optimal health, by knowing the value of health, and by coaching it and claiming it.

I want to encourage and champion a more intuitive guideline and a purposeful meaning to everyone's health and life by making a massive imprint in what they are born to do.

Anything that belongs in the health industry, which keeps us sick or makes us sicker, will not be able to survive if we all take better responsibility and ownership, and teach that to our young. We all need to make a stand, not by holding mass marches and disrupting things, but by first working on ourselves. This way is more sustainable and powerful than protests and mass marches. The latter just gives fuel to media, with an increase in opportunistic reporting that also then provides others content to put up, and round and round it goes. This content is not new but repurposed, losing its original intention and meaning, and instead giving rise to falseness and conspiracy. Pull the cord! Remember that. If we starve the crap of oxygen, do we all have a better chance to source what is true and meaningful to us? We will again be forced to go backwards.

If you think about it, how can the dieting industry, the food and agriculture industry, and the pharmaceutical industry make money from healthy people, and how can they survive if we say no to medications and to the constant treadmill of prescriptions given to us, keeping us reliant and sick? We can all reduce the consumption of targeted low-cost consumables, food, and drink that add to our problems. Instead, let's drive down the costs of good, fresh, plastic-free, organic foods so that everyone gets a chance to eat well on their budgets. I want doctors to understand the importance of organic and locally-sourced nutrition and holistic ways, prescribing guidance and advice on lifestyle, and challenging enough to get their patients listening and engaged. I know this work has begun, and it is so exciting and so needed today, for a better tomorrow for everyone.

Community doctors and healthcare professionals can learn to be champions. I have experienced a mixed bag with them, some doing some wonderful work with great care and service, and others who have sold their soul to the devil. The outcomes are that customer care is very poor, and their attitude is even worse. Let's all come away from the fact that "state" is free, and means that they can do what they want and how they want it, where patients experience the worst it has been, and kids are treated in schools in a way that goes back to the dark ages. They may as well call schools military camps, or the less abrupt would call them "free childcare camps." We all have a voice, so let's use it. Why not expect the best and help people to be the best?

I recently saw a wonderful thread on one of my social media channels, on education and how we can bring out the best in each of us, in service of these wonderful children; and many comments were positive and uplifting—the only ones that were negative were from teachers and staff of schools, blaming lack of resources. That's the emerging problem; it is always about someone else to blame, and our children are in the middle of that. If they were to think about and actually appreciate things exactly as they are, they would realise that they have a classroom to teach from, a working kitchen is available for their breaks, including a lunch break; so for a while, they can recharge. There is a staff room in which to be social with their colleagues, and they get paid every month without fail, yet they moan about the lack of resources. The only resource I see missing with many working people's ethics, is a lack of love and heart and a giving attitude. There are teachers in third world countries that would most likely crush you with their skills and their pure joy of teaching with the tiniest of resources. They get paid very little, but the children in their care are the happiest, with a "can do" attitude that far surpasses anything I have experienced with kids in the UK. They don't waste time creating behaviour policies that are so unrealistic and so controlling that so many people choose instead to homeschool—they know how more important it is to build a child rather than to take them apart. As a teacher, is that not your legacy—to build them up with confidence and a kind attitude? Are you not the role model for this, or is it all down to parents and grandparents? Some children come to school for love because they lack it at home. It is for everyone to help them, but what happens is that they get passed around social care services and have to grapple with different personalities, abilities, and motivation. This is exactly like a person/patient having a multitude of illnesses and seeing three or more physicians, with no joined-up plan to really help the human being in front of them, each only taking care of their own specialty. It is time to change this! Enough is enough. You are most likely to last longer if you take an example from those teachers that do their work from heart; and if you have never experienced it like I have, go travel to those parts of the world, and open your eyes and heart once again. Stop hiding behind government control, between conservative and labour, between republicans and democrats, where no policy or mandate is ever going to be ideal. That has to be created by you, for you, and from within yourself. You can create your world if you really want to. I saw a quote somewhere: "The right wing and left wing belong to the same bird."

You will know what it is like to be next to happy, energetic people, as opposed to tired, withdrawn, cumbersome people. It's so hard to be with people who constantly moan, criticise, and blame. No thank you! For me, my blessing is that I can intuitively gauge people's energy when I first meet them. For my clients, because they are carrying so much uncertainty in their lives, I understand that energy can be heavy, but once they start coaching, that shifts naturally and brings a huge relief to them. That, I am skilled to do, but when it comes to personal friends and colleagues, even business colleagues, their energy can be quite revealing, and I can manage myself in their company rather than be drawn into their darkness. So the trick is not to ignore or dismiss them; always be polite and kind, but what you know about how they make you feel, is enough knowledge to better manage yourself. Remember, I said that your emotional intelligence is crucial for your better navigation in life; that also means keeping the company of good people. In most cases, it does not matter to me how they dress, how wealthy they are, or how much cash they flash; I am always interested in their innocent beauty hidden deep down. Get this one thing and make peace with it: Not everyone can change, or like you. Many people in my life have come and gone. Some could not stay, not because I was bad to them or them with me, but because they could not be in the company of truth. They sought others that would not threaten them in any way. Truth is uncomfortable for many who are not ready, and what it will take for them to be ready is not for any of us to say. I remember this from some healing work I was involved with a few years back, where addicts would have to hit rock bottom before they could rise or better themselves. I hope it does not take you hitting rock bottom before you can help yourself in what you need to do, but if that is generally the direction you are going in with your life and health, make a conscious effort to hit STOP.

Back to the company of people, I have a few personal friendships with people who also live by their truth and have faced their demons, and they are much better—they are more open, and they lead their lives with heart and honesty and compassion.

Imagine how being free and open enough to positive change would feel, changes that would allow enjoyment of your life to its optimum. People like that gravitate toward each other, and people who cannot be like that, won't even try. They can't understand the divine, pure soul, and won't be able to relate to its value. Sure, they may criticise, try to control, and use all within their power to bring you down. They may even feel threatened from an ignorance perspective—let them. We have to concentrate on being free and open; others like us will gravitate toward us, and we will gravitate toward them, and the co-existence of such relationships is true joy.

We know how sport or music can transcend people's differences and abilities, and how it can bring people together for a common aim—so can health, for everyone. We have to know health fully and optimally before we know anything else. It is our foundational stake in the ground, and everything above it and to the side of it. It is an opportunity for you to be the best at what you want. So live your legacy, and impact others while you live. Let health be your signature, and join hands and hearts with others all over our beautiful planet, with this gift of and to life.

Question for you:
"Have you decided what your legacy for health is—
how you are going to live it and lead by its example?"

Guiding principle:
"We can all create a world where we are free from the burden
of ill health and preventable disease—overeating in one part of
the world, and undernourishment and famine in another—so let's
create this world by starting with one person at a time."

A New Empowering Cognitive Blueprint on Health to Pass On

We have all been in that state where we made a choice in something and then didn't understand why. When reading the book by Stephen R. Covey, *The 7 Habits of Highly Effective People,* he illustrated the example of someone's dad, who made the choice of spending time with his son instead of heeding the call to go to work. He said that his work would be there, but the time with his son would pass too quickly. His son, in that moment, felt so important, and he felt so much love and gratitude.

Putting people first and cherishing them is fundamental. With your health on your side, it is easy. It feeds a loop of feeling better in yourself and wanting to do good, with unselfish intentions self- feeding a loop into knowing right from wrong. I get goosebumps, and a lump in my throat, whenever I think of similar times when I had made those same choices, like this dad did. As a single parent with so much responsibility for so much, those choices were never ideal, but I chose to be with the kids, and I learnt to motivate them to work in our team so that I could free myself up to show up to important work and clients without feeling guilty or insufficient. The whole difficult but blessed journey meant that I was able to breathe good vibrations into every cell that exists inside me, breathing life, meaning, and purpose into it. Our human existence is truly unique.

It is a gift we don't really appreciate until something happens. When I think about all the times that people put things off that were urgent, but not important enough, because they were chasing their tails for someone else's benefit, which really had no place in their heart over the things that were so important but not urgent, like their wife or husband, their children, or even themselves. Their families were patient, and they unconditionally loved them and had learnt to tolerate the lack of their attention and time. It makes my heart heavy, but I know that not everyone has the same resources or inner strength, and that they can feel like they have no choice, but if that is a genuine situation, then correct it by giving yourself love, not guilt or a feeling of lack. For those of you who put yourself through things that are unimportant, because you can't face letting others down, you will continually let yourself down. There is always a way; we have to become creative and mindful to it. If you don't, then ask yourself what the impact of this will be on your health, as you can't turn back time.

Whose scripts are you playing out in your life? Is it even your life anymore?

Ask yourself. Seek the truth.

Whatever you are, whatever has happened, it's okay; there is great wisdom if you learn to listen, wherever you are in your journey.

So stop!

Evaluate!

Imagine that this is your last hour on earth, and your loved ones are all around you, and they have asked you to make a choice because they have a gift for you.

The choices are:

You say good-bye, and that's the end. The music and dance of your life comes to an untimely end!

Or,

You have the gift of being reborn immediately, without exit, having corrected all the things you are now aware of and wise to, and that you get this amazing chance to re-prioritise, and be more proactive and serious about your own health, as well as everything else in which you could have done better and wanted another chance to bring all things important to you into perfect balance and harmony.

What is the reason you are facing such an untimely, imminent death? Stress, cutting corners with your nutritional eating? Did you not take the signs seriously enough, despite advice and loved ones trying to get through to you? What was it? Don't lie; be very clear, and take responsibility. Do you think yourself unconquerable? Are you trying to be a martyr-type person?

Is there anyone else following your ways, and you wish something else for them because you know better?

All this information matters; look inside. It matters what you do now, and how you think and react. This is your chance.

Maybe, for some of you, this is your final chance. Only you can decide. Time is literally running out.

As they say, take the bull by its horns, and let's do this.

What is your own cognitive blueprint for your life that you want to live, and the legacy that you want to create in your world?

I know what mine is. Will you join me in creating a better and healthier world, starting with yourself?

With love and admiration, from me to you.

If you are curious as to my own experience with ill health and recovery, how I lost it and found it again, and my motivation for it in our world, then go to www.JourneyIntoRealHealth.com for a video extract that may resonate with you further.

Question for you:
"Will you join me in creating a healthier and better world?"

Guiding principle:
"The blueprint for health is in our maker;
you are one being, and we are one together."

Chapter principle:
"We can all have a healthy, happy life and live well into our old age, fully resonating with all that life has to offer in its full glory. Look after yourself. Let's look after each other. This means you will be around for longer, living fully in a wholesome and remarkable way. Make your health your legacy. It is that simple."

Printed in Great Britain
by Amazon

82654909R00241